Praise for *From OY to JOY*

From Oy to Joy is a heartwarming companion offering practical wisdom and a dose of laughter for life's challenging journey into the next chapter of life. A must read for those seeking to embrace life's transition with open hearts, open minds, and open arms.

—**John Gray,** Author, *Men are From Mars,*
Women are From Venus series,
New York Times Bestseller for five years,
Relationship Coach

I would recommend this book to anyone who wants to feel more upbeat and get encouragement for dealing with the issues of aging. — **Sheila Malkind,**
Executive Director, The Legacy Film Festival on Aging

From Oy to Joy is an enjoyable book laden with wisdom about aging and filled with practical and emotional advice, full of spirit and wisdom. — **Henry Massie, MD,**
Child and Adult Psychiatrist

A juicy, wide-opened-eyed practical guide to aging joyfully.
— **Kate Evans, PhD,**
Author

This book really helped me rise up from feeling down all the time by finding a valuable way to recognize and acknowledge unwanted changes from a new perspective. It was an "AHA" moment that helped me enjoy life more.

— **Ernestine Fields, LL.B,**
92-year-old Super Ager

From Oy to Joy is a treasure of good advice. It is full of wisdom about living a better life that, as a geriatrician, I would recommend for my patients.

— **Kenneth Covinsky, MD, MPH,**
Professor of Medicine, UCSF

While it is not easy to climb out of the prison of one's Oy orientation to aging, this book's specially designed exercises and wise suggestions, helps readers experience more of life's Joy and to expand their horizons as they grow into the next phase of their life.

— **Rabbi Stephen C. Pearce, PhD,**
Emeritus, Temple Emanuel San Franacisco

From Oy to Joy is packed with knowledge about the ups and downs of living—as a senior or indeed at any age. Especially useful in these trying times, it will make your life easier. The practical information is easily absorbed and can lead to positive changes in the reader's life.

— **Geoffrey Shaskan, PhD,**
Clinical Director, Senior Services

FROM
OY TO JOY

A Soul Journey Towards
Making the Best of Your Life
for the Rest of Your Life

Shulamit Sofia MSW

FROM OY TO JOY: A SOUL JOURNEY TOWARDS MAKING
THE BEST OF YOUR LIFE FOR THE REST OF YOUR LIFE
by Shulamit Sofia MSW

Published by
Spirit Works Press
San Francisco CA

Books can be ordered for Bulk Sales through the publisher:
spiritualaging@gmail.com

Book Design: Nick Zelinger, NZGraphics.com
Editor: Clarisa Marcee

ISBN: 978-0-9893660-2-1 (paperback)
ISBN: 978-0-9893660-3-8 (Kindle)
ISBN: 978-0-9893660-4-5 (ePub)

Library of Congress Control Number: 2024915156

First Edition

Printed in the USA

DEDICATION

To Coquelicot Gilland whose warmth, wisdom, patience, profound presence and unwavering loving support has vastly illuminated, expanded, and enriched my life

CONTENTS

The Serenity Prayer

God, grant me the serenity to accept the things
I cannot change, the courage to change the things
I can, and the wisdom to know the difference.

– Reinhold Niebuhr

FOREWORD

According to the United States Census Bureau, there are 56 million Baby Boomers, making up almost 18% of the total population, and that number is growing. *From OY to JOY: A Soul Journey to Making the Best of Your Life for the Rest of Your Life* is both timely and relevant in its wise counsel to an aging audience about how to best navigate the passage from middle age to senior status. While many consider aging as a time of loss, it actually is a time of great opportunity and a splendid gift not everyone gets to enjoy. Longevity brings with it the imperative to evolve towards a more fulfilled life of heightened wholeness. Strengthening the soul compensates in large part for the body's decline. Freedom from earlier burdens of roles and responsibilities, offers a chance, after shedding cultural and family imprints, to be able to grow into who you were always meant to be.

Aging is many things: a work in progress, a process, and especially an experience of assimilation—all of which take time, concentration, patience and especially courage. The trite saying, "Aging is not for sissies," is no joke. It is not easy but absolutely necessary to let go of what is no longer relevant to the life you had before. This book lays out the steps and strategies for shaping a more appropriate life for who you are becoming. With increasing self-awareness and authenticity, you can live an upbeat and satisfying life even when your looks fade and your strength diminishes. One such strategy is to shed what no longer serves you whether it be attitudes, thoughts, beliefs, opinions, or possessions. You learn how to dump disappointments, distress, and upset in favor of acquiring optimism, vitality, and joy.

Developing your "higher self" brings a more soulful dimension to daily life so that the stresses of the dystonic world in which we live have a lessor impact and protect you from the slings and arrows of petty pursuits. You learn how to say, "Yes" to life even when life is not saying yes to you. You learn to leave the rat race to the young who can still run it while turning your perspective inward to develop a deeper relationship with your true self, your spirit, and your soul. There is an upside to aging as you grow in soul strength and develop special skills previously not possible to pursue.

The key to graceful aging lies in moving your focus from Oy to Joy as you embark on a life of purpose. Changing your attention from the mundane to the meaningful allows you to distinguish what is authentic to you from what has been acculturated. The journey outlined in this book requires shifting from one lens to another as circumstances dictate. In the first half of life the emphasis is on your ego, the part that wants to protect you is dominant. This is necessary as you perform the adult tasks to build a career, accumulate resources, and have a family. In the second half of life, a longing for wholeness develops that must be addressed as your soul wants to heal you and make you whole, complete, and joyful regardless of the circumstances.

Discovering who you are beneath the accumulated experiences of a lifetime is the goal of longevity. Your birthright is to evolve into your authentic self, unencumbered by wanting to please others or to squeeze yourself into positions and places that don't fit who you are or who you want to become. If this is what you want to do and where you want to go, I highly recommend using this important book as your GPS in navigating your path away from Oy and towards Joy.

– Chip Conley
Modern Elder Academy founder and *New York Times* bestselling author

INTRODUCTION

"Today is the oldest you have ever been and the youngest you are ever going to be."
– Eleanor Roosevelt

Somehow when I was younger, it never occurred to me that as I grew older each year, that at some point, I would also get old. Although aware that aging was a natural, inevitable, universal process from which no one is exempt, I was totally unprepared for it actually happening to me. My awareness started in my 50s when I noticed my body was not moving with the same ease as always. In my 60s the changes accelerated, as I, like all my contemporaries, lost muscle mass and strength. I continued to exercise, take supplements, and do what I could to keep the decline at bay. In my 70s I got used to doing less and aching more. Now in my mid-80s, after happily agreeing to a long-recommended hip replacement, I am still on the go and planning to travel abroad as long as I am able. I am content with what I can do, living independently with comfort, and able to take small trips around the state. Although I have a super-ager, 79-year-old friend, by far not the youngest member of her over-70 ski club, who skied 26 times this winter, I am content to navigate as well as I do.

Although some days I ache and other days I need a nap, mostly I have the get-up-and-go to live a full life with meaning and purpose, including writing this book to share with you the skill sets I have developed along the way. This book will provide specific pointers designed to change your perspective and reframe your experience so that you can live a more joyous and fulfilled rest of your life.

While every stage of development from birth to death has its own unique challenges, aging, like adolescence, is especially demanding. Given the new and unwelcome sensations in body parts once impervious to pain, the radically different thought patterns required to successfully navigate not only this phase of life, but the brave new world in which we live, becoming an elder involves coalescing divergent evolving parts into the new person you are becoming. Add in concerns about future capacity to function at an accustomed level and the opportunities to become anxious and/or depressed multiply. By reading this book, you will learn ways of coping that will support your developing greater consciousness and mindfulness of the present moment so that you can build the necessary skills and increased awareness to be more capable of dealing with what is happening in both your external and internal environments.

Even though I am an introspective person by nature, increasing my self-awareness as well as raising my consciousness of the world around me took both practice and patience. While it was not excessively difficult, it was also by no means easy. If you are new to the process, an even greater effort will be required. As you start to walk this path it is important to be aware that things may not go as smoothly or as quickly as you would like. However, with sufficient perseverance, you will find the payoff to be enormous. There are many benefits to be gained as you learn to switch to an internal focus when needed and back when not. You will learn to experience joy by releasing expectations and judgments of how things should or should not be.

It is easy and only human to be dismayed by the unwanted changes arriving as the birthdays add up. You may feel as if the body you once took for granted is betraying you. Even worse, there is nothing you can do but grin and bear it. *From OY to JOY* was written to teach you how to grin more and bear less. It will be your road map to shifting the complaints and disappointments of an Oy-filled life to one of acceptance, appreciation, and joy.

The current structure of your life may no longer fit who you are becoming as you age. It is time to let go and allow the shifts in your immediate world to accommodate this transition. What once worked before, no longer does.

Consider that it may be time to embrace a new approach to life. Just as the caterpillar transforms into a butterfly after a period of darkness in the cocoon, so may you experience a necessary period of darkness before your new self can emerge. While I may not have attained butterfly status, I do feel that I have made major shifts in my life including moving from my previous profession to my retirement and writing this book. It has been a journey, and an example of the work one must do to have a happier old age.

Here is my story. I was the president of a non-profit organization called Caring For Children that I founded more than 36 years ago to bring emotional healing to traumatized children. This organization was the only non-profit in the world to bring solace and support to vulnerable youngsters whose lives had been disrupted without any therapy or emotional support. To help them adjust to their new circumstances, Caring For Children used the teddy bears as psychological tools to comfort the children when they were sad, lonely or afraid. More than toys the teddy bears were therapeutic objects that helped the child make a transition during a difficult time. They were an intrinsic part of our program to train their caregivers in ways of being more knowledgeable and more available to meet the children's emotional needs. My mission defined my identity, who I was, and my purpose in the world. And then, after so many years helping more than 200,000 children, it all collapsed in a matter of months due to the pandemic. The children were quarantined, the teddy bears were stuck in China, I was faced with the challenge of adapting to a more difficult reality. The alternative was to accept that it might be time to relinquish treasured goals and dreams.

A foremost task in coming to terms with one's age is the need to relinquish treasured goals and dreams that are impossible to fulfill. It is a basic hallmark of accepting old age not to persevere in pursuing activities that drain your energy without producing the desired results. In giving up Caring For Children, I had lost my vocation and my mission simultaneously and needed to recreate who I was by developing new goals that were both in alignment with the new me and possible to pursue. It was a difficult transition that led me, ultimately, to writing this book.

In summary, it was clearly time for me to release a way of life that was becoming increasingly untenable. It was apparent that I needed to reframe my vision for a future to be more in alignment with the reality of my increasing age and diminishing strength. Letting go of my treasured but impossible dream created space for new opportunities to emerge. I began to discover new ways of engaging with the world that facilitated my moving from an experience of

Oy to one of Joy. Perhaps my lesson could be yours as well. You now have a road map for shifting the complaints and disappointments of an Oy-filled life to one of acceptance, appreciation, and Joy. It will be of enormous help as you confront the many experiences and circumstances that will challenge you along the way.

You will learn new ways of being and new approaches that will ease the challenges of walking a new path to an unknown future. You will find that the journey is easier when you leave your baggage behind and learn to separate your essential self from whatever is happening around you. Even in the middle of a storm, your life can be bright and shining if you are able to engage from a place of joy. You have already started your journey by virtue of reading this now, so venture forth with confidence towards a more satisfying elder experience. Let's begin.

YOUR STARTING POINT

"Tell me, what is it you plan to do with your one wild and precious life?"
– Mary Oliver

"Life isn't about finding yourself, it's about creating yourself."
– George Bernard Shaw

You are at the beginning of a very important stage of your life with the power to shape it according to your thoughts and actions. Since they are based on your emotions and beliefs, this book will provide the opportunity to reflect, identify, and record your feelings and experiences both at the start of this process and at subsequent points along the way.

To make the most of your journey through the material presented in the book, please fully respond to the personal reflection questions at the end of each chapter in written form. You can do this directly in the book in the space provided, or you can keep a journal for this purpose.

Here are some suggestions to enable you to do just that:

- Take time to write your responses to the Personal Reflection questions as you go along.

- If you choose to answer in a separate journal, be sure to keep it with you throughout the journey of reading this book.

- Allow this process to expand your capacity to reflect on what you are learning as that will amplify what you are able to absorb and integrate.

These personal reflections will both raise your consciousness and provide you with the building blocks that create a new and more rewarding way of dealing with the life challenges and difficulties that are part of the human experience.

These Starting Point questions will establish the beginning of your trajectory of growth. Then you will have a reference point for looking back when you reach the end of this book to see how far you have come.

Personal Reflections on Your Starting Point

Describe the life you would like to live.

What would it take to achieve that?

What is the best way to move forward?

How are you holding yourself back?

What obstacles do you want to overcome?

What do you need to release (thoughts, feelings, relationships) in order to achieve your goals?

How can you become more conscious, aware, and more present in every moment?

What daily ritual or routine can you create to support your staying on track?

CHAPTER 1

ORIENTATION AND OVERVIEW

"The greatest discovery of our generation is that human beings can alter their lives by altering their attitudes of mind."
– **William James**

"Joy is not in things, it is in us."
– **Richard Wagner**

You gain wisdom as a result of your significant life experiences as well as your mistakes. As you learn to distinguish what is possible from what is not, you also learn that you can never turn back the hands of time or make people fit your expectations. However, it is totally within your power to change yourself, your perceptions, needs, and desires. You can instantly shift from Oy to Joy by changing the meaning you assign to your perceptions and experiences. Let me repeat. Change your thoughts, change your mind. Change your mind, change your life.

In the 1940s, when I was a kid, I was fascinated with the *Your Hit Parade* songs of that time, which came with printed lyrics. The song I resonated with most was "Ac-Cent-Tchu-Ate the Positive", which started with the line: "You've got to accentuate the positive, eliminate the negative, latch on to the affirmative, and don't mess with Mr. In-Between." That seemed to me to be sage advice then and still resonates now. Another song from that era "Look for the Silver Lining" echoes the same wise message. More than half a century later these sayings still ring true and present a massively effective strategy for shifting from Oy to Joy.

SHIFTING FROM OY TO JOY

Since the Oys represent a dreary mindset wherein aging is seen as a catastrophic time when aches and pains and thoughts about future disasters run rampant, it is imperative to transform that negative mindset to a more positive one. You can create joy by replacing negative thoughts with a mindset that is positive and pleasurable. Focusing on what is pleasing to you opens a door to abundant joy. To get to that place of joy requires clearing out old, outdated beliefs, opinions, and thoughts that dampen your sense of well-being. To support you in your process, this book illuminates the various debilitating thoughts, habits, and mindsets that keep you stuck on the side of Oy. This array of negative thoughts deserves a category of their own. I call this category "The

Dreadful Ds" because they always diminish your happiness and depress your sense of well-being. The Dreadful Ds to be avoided include:

- Doubt
- Discouragement
- Depression
- Disappointment
- Dysfunction
- Detachment
- Defeat
- Despair
- Deterioration
- Distancing
- Death Orientation

Your goal is to eliminate these negative influences and replace them with attributes, character traits, habits, and mindsets that constitute Your "A" Game to be described.

The Oys result from focusing on what is wrong, unwanted, and frustrating. They carry an aura of victimhood and powerlessness. You dismiss the Dreadful Ds by reclaiming your personal power. Since what you focus on expands, doesn't it make sense to focus on what you want more of and not the other way around?

Not only does the collective negativity of the Dreadful Ds diametrically oppose the qualities needed to create the life you want, but their negativity can also cause you to abandon hope for a more joyful life. As you navigate this major life transition, you must first dump all your negative thoughts and replace them with life-enhancing thoughts that support you in the years ahead.

As you read this book, you will begin to gain new awareness of yourself, others, and the world. Take the time to explore how this enhanced awareness plays out in your life. This is a good time to start the practice of journaling so you can begin to capture this new knowledge of what has been happening in your life under the surface of your consciousness. In addition to gaining new awareness of the patterns in your life from your earliest memories, you will become more conscious about how they are currently operating. You may want to return to this section after completing the book to compare what you are now understanding from having read the book to how you were before you began.

THE DREADFUL Ds

DOUBT can grow in your mind, sabotage your intention and your ability to meet your goals.

DISCOURAGEMENT comes from falsely believing that what you want is not possible when it well might be.

DEPRESSION is the end result of draining your energy and destroying your dreams.

DISAPPOINTMENT is an emotional letdown when what was wanted does not manifest. By fixating on what didn't transpire, you do nothing to change the situation, only lament it.

DYSFUNCTIONAL is that disabling and self-destructive behavior keeping you stuck.

DETACHMENT is the psychological mechanism that distances you from painful feelings of disappointment, depression, defeat, and despair.

DEFEAT is the experience of giving up on yourself and all possibilities for change.

DESPAIR is a deep, dark, depressed mood that impedes any possibility for positive action.

DETERIORATION is the result of not taking positive action on your own behalf.

DISTANCING separates you from the flow of life by withdrawing from the world, which only reinforces what you want to eliminate.

DEATH ORIENTATION is totally giving up on yourself and life itself.

At any point, you can choose to change any and all of these attitudes and attributes and reengage in ways that create new opportunities for less stress and more success.

Which of the Dreadful Ds most resonate with you?

How does this interfere with the way you live your life?

What are three steps you can take to shift this debilitating mindset?

BRING ON THE JOY BY PLAYING YOUR "A" GAME

Playing the "A" Game requires your full attention and the best of your ability. "A" Game designation is relative to each person's ability and capacity, not an external standard. You are performing at an "A" Game level when you continuously aim for your highest standards with intention and commitment. If you have been giving it your all, in terms of abilities, understanding, knowledge, perseverance, and energy, then you are a winner regardless of the results.

Your greatest challenge will be to obtain, maintain, and sustain a positive mindset and sufficient motivation to attain your goals. Especially if you have been defeated, depleted, or challenged in the past by self-doubt, low self-esteem, or pessimism, it is important to acknowledge yourself and know that you have taken all the necessary steps to get beyond your past. Never, ever give up. Your positive mindset makes all the difference. While it takes massive action to get you to where you want to go, even small steps can take you far. Just breaking the bond of inertia, in itself, can be life changing.

YOUR "A" GAME
ASTOUNDING ADMIRABLE ADVENTURES

Your "A" Game is a complex of attitudes and behaviors that allow you to develop those attributes that best support your emotional well-being and spiritual growth.

ATTITUDE is the most significant variable in your personal development. It is also the one thing totally under your control. The late Viktor Frankl, author of *Man's Search for Meaning* realized while imprisoned in a Nazi concentration camp that no matter how many of his personal freedoms were taken away, his attitude was still under his control. He later wrote, "Everything can be taken from a man but one thing: the last of human freedoms—to choose one's attitude in any given circumstances, to choose one's own way."

ALLOWING is the essential first step in relinquishing resistance to your current reality. Since what you resist persists, your first step is to recognize and allow what is present in your current reality to be what it is however unwanted it may be.

ACCEPTING is the next step of coming to terms with precisely those elements in your life that are the most difficult for you to deal with.

ACCOMMODATING is adjusting your actions and expectations to allow for new possibilities to emerge.

APPRECIATION is looking for the good in everything including things that do not appear at first to be positive knowing in the long run, it is for your best.

ADAPTABILITY involves your recognition that while you have the capacity to mold many things more to your liking, some things you cannot change no matter how hard you try. This is the time to remember "The Serenity Prayer" that teaches us to distinguish what you can change from what you cannot, and then accepting what you cannot change. Adaptability provides the flexibility to make the necessary shifts when life is unbending.

ACTION is the only way to initiate change or make progress. Once you have evaluated how to respond to the circumstances it is imperative to take action in order to produce results.

Your first step to making the best of the rest of your life is to no longer resist what you resent. Rather, remind yourself to look for whatever is good in any situation or person and teach yourself to pivot from what you don't like to what you do. By persuing this process you are engaged in building the spiritual muscle and soul strength that will sustain you as you age. Embrace the steps outlined above, continue to move in the direction of your "A" Game as best you can and stay focused on your end goal. Use the chapters to come as guideposts along the path. You can begin your journey on your own or share it with travel buddies.

As you enter the third act of your life and begin to integrate your new level of understanding and awareness on a deeper level, your long dormant spirituality begins to awaken. This enables you to put worries, doubts, distractions, and dissatisfactions into perspective. You learn to accept life as it is without the futile attempt of trying to control it since controlling life is an absolutely impossible task. Rather, it is the opposite that is called for. Only when you release your Oys along with your need to control life, can you experience the Joys. Only by accepting your life as it is can you embrace the aging process as it unfolds. Acceptance is your key to living a happier life.

CHAPTER 2

WHAT IS AGING?

*"People don't grow old. When they stop growing,
they become old."*
– Anonymous

"Aging is something that happens, if you are lucky—and it is very hard work," states a 91-year-old retired attorney who received her law degree at age 58 and didn't stop practicing until suffering a heart attack at age 89. She is absolutely correct. No matter how much one may smile when hearing the saying, "aging is not for sissies," it is not a joke. Aging, much like adolescence, is a growth process that results in creating a new identity for the person you are becoming.

This is your last opportunity to become your authentic self—knowing there are many paths to that authenticity. It takes courage to accept and adjust to the unwanted changes that arrive as the birthdays add up. With the appearance of wrinkles combined with the loss of energy, and hormonal fluctuations, you might feel as if the body you once took for granted is betraying you. It is not. It is offering you an opportunity to appreciate yourself on a deeper level.

Webster's dictionary has a dual definition of aging that sums up an essential dichotomy in a single sentence. Aging is described either as growing old or becoming mature as the two life-path options. Which one will you choose? Do you want to grow old with all the negative connotations of Oy or do you want to mature with all its possibilities for Joy? As you go forward in life, you will have to decide whether you want to age/deteriorate or to mature/blossom.

Deepak Chopra cites research to be discussed in Chapter 9 that verifies you are only as old as you think you are. That is Clint Eastwood's strategy. At 92, he states his secret is "not to let the old man in." That is my strategy as well. It is a practice I do daily. Therefore, keep thinking of yourself as young and vital. I constantly am amazed and very grateful at what I can still do at my advanced age of 85. I swim and do water aerobics three times a week, take three yoga classes a week and try to walk but don't always reach my goal of two miles a day. I recently completed a two-month solo bucket trip to six countries around the Mediterranean.

At the same time, no one is ever fully prepared for the accumulative effects of incremental changes impacting your body and impairing your functioning. Who is this stranger in the mirror? And how did all your friends and family get so old?

It takes spiritual strength and acquiring new adaptive skills in order to stay positive when your world is shifting beneath your feet. If lucky, you stumble a bit. If not so lucky, you repeatedly fall down and need to persevere in picking yourself up and keep on going.

Maturation comes from learning from the past. By gathering, assimilating, and reviewing your thoughts, beliefs, opinions, and memories of a lifetime, you are restructuring your identity from who you have been into who you are becoming. Knowing who you have been and who you have now become frees you to proceed to the next phase of your life. By releasing the parts that no longer fit, you are sculpting a new self. And the more you let go of what is no longer useful, relevant or to your liking, the more the true you emerges.

Living to a ripe old age is a very recent gift of time. We are the first generation to have lived long past roles and responsibilities. At the start of the last century, the average life expectancy was 47.8, now it's 78.9, almost double and continuing to rise. Until now, shorter lifespans precluded the opportunity to journey on the spiritual path of becoming whole and authentic. Prior to our generation's expanded lifespan, there was little time or space for personal development given the roles and responsibilities of being an adult, making a living, and rearing children.

Aging is your late-in-life opportunity to become "real,"— the person you were born to become. According to Margery Williams, author of *The Velveteen Rabbit*, "Generally, by the time you are Real, most of your hair has been loved off and your eyes drop out and you get loose in the joints and very shabby. But these things don't matter at all because once you are Real, you cannot be ugly, except to people who don't understand."

You begin your journey to Joy by letting go of expectations and attachments. As you free your mind of disappointments and other negative thoughts, you experience only those thoughts that nurture and support your psychological growth and the emerging of a more authentic self. This includes releasing enculturated societal stereotypes, cultural conditionings, and family indoctrination. Use this opportunity to uncover your true inclinations, preferences and interests and follow the path to self-fulfillment.

Most of us carry within us memories, beliefs, attitudes, stories, and emotional imprints from our childhood. Now is the time to start letting go of those parts that no longer serve you. You are not the same person you were when you made them. Recognize the need for an update. It is also time to shift your perspective from the experiences of the physical world to exploring an inner world of spirit. When you shift your focus from understanding others to understanding yourself you embark on an internal adventure of self-discovery. You have begun the adventure of spiritual aging.

Taking responsibility for your own growth is especially important in a culture like ours that denigrates and demonizes aging. Unlike other cultures where elders are integrated into extended families, honored with great respect, and revered for their wisdom, elders in our society are viewed as disposable and obsolete, moved into assisted living and nursing homes, and essentially ignored. If that is not the life you want for your later years, then you must prepare immediately for being valued, honored, and respected in old age starting with respecting yourself.

These two approaches to aging are demonstrated in the stories of two long-time friends Carole and Susan, who met in high school and despite their different personalities and divergent life experiences, maintained a warm friendship for more than 60 years. Each exemplifies a different life choice. Carole was well on the road to old age even in her thirties as she was excessively anxious and worrisome her entire life. She was always complaining and dissatisfied with her experience no matter where she was or what was happening. Unfortunately, a severe stroke in her 70s left her extremely incapacitated and in need of assisted living. She has now moved several times, finding none so far that pleased her. Susan, in contrast, had a very upbeat personality. Now 76, she is as spry as ever, traveling, enjoying a meaningful fun-filled relationship. Which of these divergent paths would you prefer?

Aging gracefully takes skill and the practice of building those skills. It's also important to know you can more easily shed the outgrown parts of yourself when you are more conscious of your inner attitudes on a deeper level. Your job is to unpeel the accumulated cultural, societal, and family imprinting and conditioning to reveal your true self. While these may have once served you, they are now detrimental to the developmental tasks of this stage of life.

How does this relate to you and your patterns of thought? It is time to understand fully the degree to which your mental state and emotional well-being is directly impacted by your thoughts and feelings. Do you know what makes you happy and what dampens your joy? Are you ready to learn to release disempowering patterns formed by your habitual thoughts and feelings? Increasing your self-knowl-edge helps you avoid what brings you down. It also helps you pay more attention to what elevates your thoughts and, thus, your mood. Avoiding what deflates your sense of well-being will automatically increase it.

By improving alignment between your essential inner self (soul) and the façade you present to the world (ego), you become more congruent and authentically self-expressive. It is important to look forward and face the future, as reliving the past only negates your efforts to create new opportunities and explore new possibilities. Your true self has been waiting decades to emerge from its self-imposed exile. Don't waste time and energy better spent creating a new tomorrow. Do not let the past distract you. The only path that matters is the one facing forward. The reason the rear-view mirror is so small is so it does not obscure the view forward.

Your road to a more joyous life starts with changing your thoughts. Change your thoughts, change your mind. Change your mind, change your life.

Many elders have shown us the way to live a vibrant life well into old age. They too had to create a workable way of facing an uncertain future in unfamiliar territory. They learned it takes more courage and ingenuity to deal with decline than it does to deal with growth. Gloria Steinem described the challenges of aging as akin to visiting a foreign country where you have never been before, where you don't know any of the street names, nor directions to any of that country's most interesting places. Nor do you know how to speak the language, but it still feels like a fabulous adventure awaits you. Only when she surrendered to that adventure did she begin to figure it out and if she could, so can you.

Both Lawrence Ferlinghetti, a renowned San Francisco Beat Poet, and Betty White, the cherished TV star, are examples of those who were able to remain professionally active while nearing their 100th birthdays. Another sterling example is Queen Elizabeth who at age 96, only two days before her death, was fulfilling her role as sovereign of Great Britain by swearing in a new Prime Minister. Jane Fonda, Helen Mirren, and Rita Moreno are all past 80 looking gorgeous and still performing. Also going strong is Pope Francis who continues traveling the world in his wheelchair bringing love and hope to multitudes. Recently, I interviewed an incredible 94-year-old woman for this book who is still traveling, although no longer alone (she gave that up at 89) and said, "Next time I go to the airport, I think I will get a wheelchair."

Personal Reflections

On a scale of one to ten, how comfortable are you with the aging process?

Which aspects do you find the most challenging?

How do you deal with the Dreadful Ds and worries about the future?

Which habits of thought or behavior can you eliminate?

What steps can you take to eliminate them?

What thoughts and habits can you replace them with?

What models do you have in your life that demonstrate graceful aging?

What specifically could you learn from them to include in your life?

If you have no model, look for one in the culture. Describe.

What resources do you need to gather to facilitate your staying on track as you begin your journey to building the soul strength to age spiritually as well as physically?

What kind of routine can you establish that would give you the structure required for successfully navigating a soul journey?

Who or what can you utilize to support your success in developing your "A" Game?

CHAPTER 3

SPIRITUAL AGING

"Age is not a problem to be solved or a challenge to overcome but an opportunity for a new level of spiritual maturity."
– Carol Orsborn

Your spiritual approach to aging begins when concerns about physical appearance and the opinions of others are replaced with deeper issues of character and the power higher than yourself. Suddenly, you are no longer interested in acquiring and achieving more. Rather, you are inspired to start shedding your excess material possessions and attachments. You feel safer and more satisfied when in tune with your spiritual side. This is no easy task in a culture dominated by an emphasis on material success. It takes considerable inner work to value not what we have materially, but who we are on our deepest level.

Growing up in a capitalistic culture teaches you to worship money and power not humanitarian values such as humility, kindness, or generosity. Have you succumbed to the myth that money buys happiness? Even when you know that it does not, the momentary pleasure and/or distraction it provides from emotional and psychological pain, makes it important. However, money can never truly bring you peace of mind and a life of joy. Instead, the higher self with its more elevated interests, activities, and virtues needs to be engaged and encouraged. Aging offers an opportunity to reexamine your values and to determine where to look for happiness.

In spiritual terms we all have two selves. The first self, the small self, called ego is totally concerned with your safety in order to ensure your physical and psychological survival. This small self is an absolutely necessary part of your makeup. Its job is to protect you at all times. Unfortunately, ego, in our society, is in overdrive, anxious about succeeding in its perceived job of protection. Ego is where your fears and anxiety reside and where you get easily triggered. It is impossible to be joyous when the ego is in charge because it is always on high alert, easily threatened by life circumstances, and needs to feel in control in order to feel safe. It constantly scans the environment for evidence of danger. At one time, survival in a primitive world filled with physical dangers required such vigilance. A tiger might pop up at any time. However, now that pattern leads to pervasive anxiety about your well-being.

Your ego now interferes with the emergence of your higher self by perceiving threats where none exist.

This is not to say there are not real dangers to your physical well-being in this time of economic insecurity, health threats, rising urban violence, and extreme weather. However, while it's necessary to be savvy in how you conduct yourself outside your home, it is also important for your peace of mind to reduce your concerns to a minimum. Most important is developing a sense of safety within yourself by learning to trust that you will be safe and secure regardless of what is going on around you. That is an essential part of the voyage from Oy to Joy.

Your other self is your higher self, or soul, which is concerned about your development as a person with emphasis on your character, your integrity, and your place in the universe. Your higher self or soul connects you to a power greater than yourself. Focusing on your soul, or higher self, is the essence of spiritual aging. The material outer world diminishes in attraction as you turn your gaze to your inner world of a yet-to-be-discovered self. Your soul's mission is to connect you with the larger universe of all that is, the place of all creation where you and your ego are but a tiny speck. Your concern is no longer with status, possessions, or recognition. Dr. Robert Grant, author of *The Way of the Wound* writes, "All forms of spirituality are rooted in not living exclusively for oneself from an ego dominated consciousness." He adds, "To be touched by spirit is to discover a fuller participation in ordinary living."

Moving towards a more spiritual orientation will enhance your life as you develop the soul strength and resiliency that bolsters your ability to cope with the adverse vicissitudes of life. Your ego will protest as its influence shrinks and the problems of the material world take second place to the development of your inner life. The strengthening of your soul more than compensates for the discomfort of this transition. This process of building spiritual muscle uses the adversity you experience and the challenges you face as building blocks to develop soul strength. It is a process by which you are transformed from your survival self to your higher self. Like building physical musculature it takes commitment, consistency, and character to do the necessary many reps.

The steps laid out in the following material enable you to elevate your ingrained or conditioned behavior by learning the techniques that enable to deal more effectively with the unfair, unwanted, and unfavorable challenges with equanimity and peace of mind. The more you practice, the easier it gets, but keep in mind that it is never easy.

As you become better prepared to deal with the challenges of aging, both psychologically and physically, you will be less likely to restrict your life by focusing on adverse factors. Academic research has documented that worrying is detrimental to your health. In fact, it can cost you on the average of 7.5 more years of life according to Yale University researcher Dr. Becca Levy who found a correlation between more positive attitudes and better health and longevity. More dramatically, researchers at Bar-Ilan University followed nearly 200 patients ages 73-84 who had a variety of conditions from fractures to strokes. They found those who felt youngest at admission, regardless of their actual age, made the best progress and showed greater functional independence at discharge regardless of condition. They also found that subjective age was a stronger predictor to rehabilitation outcomes than either chronological age or chronic health conditions.

Spiritual muscle helps you stay positive in the face of unwanted changes in your body. Building spiritual muscle is what you will be learning as you travel through this book. It is a path I am traveling as well. I have become significantly more challenged, as in the course of writing this book I have acquired more medical concerns along the way. Needless to say, I do not like the new findings but, since resistance is futile, I have embraced them. The gift of spiritual aging is its perspective on how to live a happier and more fulfilling old age.

You begin or accelerate an inner journey strengthened by trust in a higher power. Your view of your life changes as you increasingly realize that you are not your body but rather a transcendent soul housed in a physical form. You shift your perspective in other ways as well. Your concerns about the outer world diminish as the dynamics of your inner landscape increase. Beyond concerns about the physical signs of your body changing, you are more interested in what is happening on the deepest level of your being. Weight on your physical form becomes less an issue than the heaviness in your heart. A society alienated from its soul, where the prevailing belief is that only what can be sensed is real, does not recognize this dichotomy. As you progress on your spiritual path and begin to see yourself in a new perspective, you increasingly realize the tenuousness of all existence and that at the deepest level you are but a fleeting speck in a massive universe.

Therefore, allow your soul's desires to guide you rather than following your ego's fears. This approach frees you from ego domination and alleviates anxiety. As you are able to relax into feeling you have "enough," you can relax your excessive striving to accumulate more in the material world. That is a game without end. You will never be satisfied, feel secure, or experience success as long as you continue striving for more. A young stockbroker once told me, "It was only when I began to accumulate considerable wealth and was exposed to people who were mega-rich, that I began to feel poor." How perverse is that?

As you age, you increasingly want to simplify your life and release possessions rather than accumulate more. In fact, one indication that you are living a spiritual life is a growing disinterest in having more "things." Another indication is increased equanimity regarding the visible signs of your aging. You now have the ability to accept these changes as an inevitable part of the life process. You can now view yourself through the more valuable lens of your own personal integrity and become indifferent to how others judge you. Being true to yourself becomes a more substantial question than how you look. As you let go of strenuous efforts to maintain a more youthful appearance, you can allow yourself to be guided by your soul's desires, rather than your ego's fears. You are more present in the moment without looking back to the past or forward to the future. You no longer define your personal success by contemporary social standards. Most important, you learn to be compassionate towards yourself, with all your imperfections. All through my life I was painfully aware of my self-perceived inadequacies and was always striving to correct them. I wanted to be more organized, more competent in my decisions, more put together in my appearance. I was always striving to move towards a moving target I could never reach. Now I am interested in being more patient, more tranquil, more loving in my responses to myself and others.

Spiritual aging is a process where who you are on the inside is more important than how you look on the outside. When you stop identifying with your body and your ego's narrow self-interest, you enter a more expansive world where alternative pathways open in the direction of your dreams. As your perceptions, and the meaning you assign to them change, you are able to open your eyes to a new perspective. Like any journey, there will be ups and downs requiring patience, persistence and faith. Be strong and persevere until the evidence of change becomes apparent as you better adapt to the new circumstances of your life. It is a lifelong journey to become who you are on the deepest level of your authentic self.

Self-discovery and carving your own path to your desired future and full self-expression is your ultimate task in this aging adventure. Following are some strategies from among many spiritual practices able to lead you to where you want to go. As the power of your ego diminishes, following these practices will amplify your ability to be in tune with your inner wisdom.

Reaching your higher self includes the following practices:

MEDITATION

Meditation is a fundamental practice that opens a portal to your inner world. Your deepest thoughts become more accessible as you learn to quiet your monkey mind. Distracting random thoughts fade with time as your ability to focus becomes stronger with practice. Learning to still your mind begins by focusing on something available to your senses. One traditional way to begin is to stare at a candle or notice your breath as it goes in and out. As your breath slows down, so does your mind. Even a short daily practice leads to greater self-awareness on a deeper level. As you begin letting go of disruptive thoughts, greater stillness and new levels of awareness will soon become available to you.

Patterns of thoughts, feelings, and behaviors to which you were previously oblivious become more apparent the longer you meditate. Even a five-minute practice period in the morning and five minutes in the evening will yield considerable results. Extending practice periods produces more peace of mind and less anxiety. Be aware, the pump needs priming, so be prepared to practice for some period of time before the flow begins.

For those who find it hard to sit still, a walking meditation may be more to your liking. A meditation walk is carefully choreographed with each component simplified and slowed down. Every step is carefully articulated to consist of slow partial steps and long pauses. You begin with your hands folded and held heart-level at your chest. Start by taking a deep breath and balancing on one foot; take one very slow partial step with the other. Stop. Pause. Wait. Breathe. Then slowly take the next part of the step. Repeat. Keep repeating.

Because a meditative process is not only fundamental to spiritual growth but also essential to coming to terms with the existential anxiety of dealing with the unfamiliarity of change, you may be urged to turn to meditation many times while reading this book.

BREATHING

Breathing is so fundamental to life that without your constant breathing you have no life. Furthermore, the deeper you breathe the more alive your body becomes. You can alter your state, elevate your mood, and improve your mental status with a conscious breathing practice pattern. You can even increase your energy level and create a sense of calm by doing breathing exercises. There are numerous valuable formulas for breathing patterns with various combinations of inhales, exhales, and holds. One basic breathing sequence that is easy to follow suggests inhaling for four counts, holding it for a count of six, and breathing out to the count of eight. Another common practice is "box" breathing with an inbreath to the count of four, a hold of four, and an outbreath of four. The discipline and structure of a regular practice will provide both extra oxygen intake as well as a release of toxins as air is dispelled through the long exhale. The increased oxygen on the inhale with the release of toxins when breathing out enhances brain function. You will soon feel better and even think better.

BEING IN NATURE

One of the most pleasant of the practices suggested is to be in nature. The natural world is a tonic that calms your nervous system and helps keep you grounded and present in the moment. Simply sitting is relaxing and soothing, but walking outside, especially barefoot on grass or sand, is preferable. It relaxes your whole body and amplifies your well-being. You may want to explore some books and/or some products that promote grounding with earth energy nourishment.

SENSING

This fundamental practice requires being quiet while becoming purposefully hyper-aware of external and internal stimuli. When you slow down sufficiently to expand your field of awareness, then you can notice, like the biblical Moses, that which is not readily apparent to others. With a sufficient level of concentration, you too can become aware that the burning bush was not being consumed. You can also learn to be sensitive to your own body and develop awareness of where tension is stored in your body, how your posture impacts your sense of well-being, and how various foods impact your energy level. This increased awareness makes you more sensitive to and engaged with usually unnoticed aspects of your daily life.

SACRED TEXTS

Sacred texts are inspirational and feed both your mind and your soul by elevating your consciousness with noble thoughts. When read in a class or other group setting, not only is this activity emotionally nourishing in itself, but it also provides the social connections so vital to combating feelings of loneliness and isolation in old age.

PERSONAL PRAYER

Prayer, the process of communicating with a higher power from your heart, can be extremely comforting and soothing. As a daily ritual it can quickly transport you to a place of peace and calm. There are three basic types of prayer. The first level is petitionary prayer, which is asking God for something whether it be more money, a new car, a healthier body, or some improved circumstance of life. At the next level are thankfulness prayers expressing generalized gratitude and appreciation for already answered prayers. At the highest level are the prayers of praise, called Hallel, from which the word Hallelujah, which means praise God in Hebrew, is formed.

Personal Reflections

On a scale of one to ten, how religious was the home you grew up in?

How spiritual was the home you grew up in?

How religious are you now?

How spiritual are you now?

On a scale of one to ten, how strong is your ego orientation to life? Describe.

On a scale of one to ten, how strong is your higher self orientation to life? Describe.

Which one do you feel more comfortable with?

Which spiritual practices resonate most?

Which spiritual practices support your enhanced sense of well-being?

Describe how this is expressed in your mindset and behavior.

CHAPTER 4

CHASING AWAY THE OYs

"Keep your face to the sunshine and you will never see the shadows."
– Helen Keller

Although the Oys often come to visit, they only remain if the guardian of the gate of your mind allows them to stay. You can choose to entertain only the visitors you want, and the rest are politely turned away. While it is human nature to doubt and ruminate about what might have, could have, should have been done differently, it is your choice whether or not to pay attention to such compulsive and intrusive thoughts. Such ideation is simply not useful and often harmful. Since you are perfectly free to choose another channel, it is time to train yourself to dismiss those daily capricious thoughts crossing your mind. As you assume responsibility for being the editor of your mind's content, your ability to regulate the thoughts that populate your consciousness grows stronger. You learn to preserve what enhances your experience and ignore the rest. You will notice over time that the neural pathways of dismissed negative thoughts grow weaker with disuse, thus making it easier for you to enjoy a more positive and peaceful state of mind.

A major source of Oy is dealing with regrets and other remnants of unfinished business. It is often easy for you to lose control of your resolve to move forward when a flood of emotions, triggers, sensitivities, and the residue of earlier trauma provoke a regressive response. It is of utmost importance not to give these thoughts your energy or attention. Rather, keep your mind clear and your eyes on the prize.

MANAGING YOUR THOUGHTS

There are many methods for managing your thoughts. Following are a few I use.

SUBSTITUTION

Choosing and concentrating on positive thoughts that substitute for unwanted negative ones not only reinforces positive thinking but spares you from the negative impact of thoughts not beneficial to your well-being. It is easy to doubt yourself and feel unworthy of accomplishing a task or receiving a reward. Don't fall into that pattern. As Henry Ford so famously stated, "Whether you think you can, or you think you can't, you are right." Every time your doubt comes up, remind yourself that you can. Each time when I told myself "I don't know how," I had to rephrase that into I can learn, find out, or hire a consultant.

PERSPECTIVE

Another way to change your thoughts is to change your perspective. I learned in art school when drawing a still life placed in the center of the room that no student has the exact same view. You literally see things only from where you stand. Your goal is to be aware of these differences and acknowledge them. Respect another person's point of view. It does not make it wrong because it is not the same as yours. I learned another aspect about perspective many years ago in San Francisco while with friends watching the approaching sunset over the Pacific Ocean. When my companion pointed out how absolutely gorgeous the sun setting over the water was, I responded, "Yes, except for those ugly wires spoiling the view." His profound yet simple reply was, "Turn your head and you won't see them anymore." Those wise words have stayed with me ever since and remind me that it is always possible to change your perspective.

HYPERFOCUS

Sometimes the opposite of dismissing your thoughts is also effective. By intensifying your attention to and exaggerating unwanted thoughts, either by consciously repeating them in your mind or repeatedly speaking them aloud, you become more cognizant of what is occurring in your mind. Intentionally exaggerating the negativities that concern you enables you to objectively examine them from a detached point of view. You can also ask yourself, "Is that true?" or "How can I verify that thought?" Then, from that perspective, you can decide if your thoughts make sense, are true, or are even worthy of your attention.

CEASE JUDGING YOURSELF AND OTHERS

Nothing will deflate your sense of well-being faster than critical thoughts about yourself and/or others. The more such thoughts linger, the harder it is to rid yourself of them. If you keep ruminating over them like a tongue searching out a sore tooth, they will continue to hold your attention. However, with intention and consistent practice, you will soon be able to pivot to more positive mental content. For instance, instead of determining you did not make a good presentation, ask yourself which parts did satisfy you. Better yet, ask a colleague or friend what their opinion was. Most likely they will judge you less harshly than you judge yourself. Similarly, rather than seeing the faults in another person, search for their good points. The more you practice, the more you build the necessary spiritual muscle to monitor and redirect your thoughts.

DISTRACTION

Another technique to avoid thinking about what upsets you is by consciously thinking about something else. Keeping yourself busy with another more positive activity is another way of making deposits in your emotional bank account available for later withdrawal. Excellent choices would be reading an absorbing book, learning a new language, or listening to music that transports you away from your preoccupation. Doing a creative activity such as a craft project or making a painting are among your many choices for beneficial distractions. Focusing on a positive activity is a pleasant distraction that also builds your spiritual muscle.

PHYSICAL ACTIVITY

Being physically active is not only energizing but stimulates endorphins, which, in turn, generate good feelings that will enable you to deal more effectively with negative feelings. There is much to choose from. In addition to low-impact activities like swimming, tai chi, and yoga, and Zumba Gold for seniors, there are many online classes of simple repetitive floor and wall exercises available for your choosing that promise to strengthen and tone even seniors more sedentary than you. For those who can still run around but find tennis too demanding, the new Pickleball craze delivers an opportunity to get exercise and companionship simultaneously.

CREATIVITY

This category allows you to use your mind as a diversion. There is so much to choose from including packaged activities of needle work and painting by number for those who prefer something more structured. Other options include journaling or joining a writing group. Check out your local community center where choices such as ceramics and painting may also be available. The more limber can also participate in a dance class. All these activities offer an effective form of diversion from the disheartening Oys. Instead, allow yourself the satisfaction of expressive activities that are also productive mood enhancers that support and sustain your sense of well-being by blocking obsessing and ruminating thoughts leading towards no productive end.

AWARENESS AND OBSERVATION

Being vigilant about your thoughts supports your greater self-awareness and greater peace of mind. As Shakespeare once wrote, "Nothing is good or bad but thinking makes it so." As you gain awareness and maintain a neutral position without judging or evaluating your experiences, situations, or others you avoid polluting your mind. You benefit both your brain and body by enjoying the beauty of nature.

You can do this by walking in flower gardens and greenery, strolling along the beach, or picnicking on the grass. Learn to observe without making what you are viewing either right or wrong, better or worse than something else. Increasingly seeing the beauty in the world around you feeds your soul. You wouldn't allow garbage to fill your home. Why would you allow it to fill your consciousness?

SPECIAL CHALLENGES

Since the pandemic, so much has changed and rarely for the better. There have been many challenges including increased negativity and fear, and especially digitalization of so many aspects of our life that eliminate human contact. In addition, especially for seniors, there are reduced opportunities for socialization.

The Atlantic Magazine recently published an article about how people are not hanging out together at the same levels and in the same ways they did prior to the pandemic. Life has become more difficult to navigate. In many ways, it is easier to retreat at home and not deal with any of the stresses of the outside world. At the same time, it is important to fight inertia. Staying active for as long as you can is crucial because "if you don't use it, you will lose it," a saying attributed to motivational speaker Les Brown. Sitting is now being seen as the new smoking. Be advised of the need to keep moving on a daily basis. Movement is increasingly prescribed for those who want to maintain and sustain mobility and mental agility. Don't stop swimming if you do and please start if you don't. Swimming is a marvelous way to keep your muscles stretched with less effort than doing similar exercises on land.

Older folks also face special challenges due to their fears of the future. These include:

ANXIETY ABOUT GETTING SICK

Since body parts do have an expiration date, there is a good chance that sooner or later, you are going to experience a breakdown of some kind or other. However, that does not mean that it is inevitable or that you will become ill or disabled. There is no reason to worry in advance about something that is not happening and perhaps never will. For example, instead of lamenting muscle loss, you begin to include in your practice routines that build muscle strength. Lifting weights however light is one strategy to turn your concern into appropriate activities that will retard or prevent the occurrence of the problems that worry you.

MEDIA NEGATIVITY

It is the job of media to be sensational and create fear so that people will stay tuned. The longer you remain engaged, the more profitable it is for them. Your job is to resist wasting your time following the news and social media when it could be used more productively. You can always stay informed without exposing yourself to sensationalized news designed to make you fearful and addicted. A quick scan of the headlines, watching news on your computer, or a brief conversation with a neighbor similarly committed to a news fast should keep you apprised of the most important facts.

DIVISIVENESS

In this time of great cultural division, with constant exposure to socially unacceptable behavior, it is best to abstain from conversations and other situations that are not peaceful or enhancing. It is best to avoid social media and news that engages people by getting them upset about political issues. Rather, focus on the things we share in common. Whenever possible strive for agreement or common ground. If that is not possible, gracefully absent yourself from the situation or conversation.

ANGER AND VIOLENCE

The pandemic had a huge impact on mental health issues of much of the population. The rise in incidents of violent or socially inappropriate behavior has escalated. Levels of anger and angry "acting out" behavior in vulnerable people has skyrocketed dangerously. Aggressive incidents on airplanes have tripled. Remember their unacceptable words and behavior are about them and have no relevance to you unless you allow it. Do not take anything personally and do not get triggered and react inappropriately. Protect yourself by avoiding any possible situation or conversation that could become contentious and removing yourself immediately from situations likely to get out of control.

OTHER PEOPLE'S NEGATIVITY AND ANXIETY

Since feelings are contagious, the negativity of another person can be as infectious as any virus. Protect yourself from exposure by distancing as much as you would for someone who had COVID-19. Recently, I went to an evening event on a quiet Sunday and parked in an area that had a city sign designating hours for parking without penalty. On my return from an enjoyable evening in a good mood, I was surprisingly accosted by an angry doorman from a nearby hotel who walked several yards to accuse me of having parked on hotel property. He told me he could have called the police and warned me not to do it again. Although the law was on my side, because I did not want to prolong the contention by pointing out the city sign or engaging in conversation, I simply said, "Thank you for not doing so" and left.

DEPRESSION

It is easy to be pulled down by the problems of the world and the traumas of those struggling to adapt to this rapidly changing new world. In addition to the news, which seems to get worse on a daily basis, everyone has personal problems of one kind or another that can be depressing if you are not vigilant. Your job is to stop giving such negativity your attention. You can protect yourself by using the following antidotes.

ANTIDOTES

The following activities and actions can help you cope with stress:

SIMPLE PLEASURES

The range of possibilities is unlimited, trimmed only by personal preferences. Begin to do or do more of whatever floats your boat. It's time to buffer your downside with upside energy. What that might be has enormous variation as each of us has personalized preferences. Even though there are cat people and dog people, almost everyone can agree it would be nice to have a pet to cuddle when they are feeling lonely while those who are trying to make their lives simpler don't want to take on the responsibility involved.

For those who don't want to commit to that level of care, there are other choices. One option is to have an aquarium because fish can be engaging in their own way and require less care. And you only need to give them a little food and clean their bowl. Plants need only occasional attention and contribute health benefits.

Another source of pleasure would be to take yourself on a play date. It is so much fun to indulge yourself in doing something that brings you joy when you have the impulse and the permission. What would be satisfying and stimulating for you? There are art and other types of classes at most community centers from which you can get inspiration to do things on your own outside of class. I like to explore a new neighborhood, have tea in a fancy place with a friend or visit an art museum. It is sometimes nice to do it solo and always enhanced when shared with friends. If you are homebound, perhaps you can invite people to visit you or include you in Zoom conversations. If there is an activity that really lights up your life, perhaps you can form an interest group.

GETTING SUFFICIENT SLEEP

It is during sleep that your body repairs and rejuvenates. The recommended "dose" is usually eight hours in order for you to be rested and restored. What is sufficient sleep for you? It might sometimes be more than eight hours and sometimes less. Having sufficient energy during the day is of utmost importance to live a full and productive life. Therefore, organize your bedtime in ways you can prepare for a good night's sleep. Start by winding down before bedtime. You do that by turning off the TV before 10:00 pm, and putting away, preferably in a different room, your cell phone and other electronic devices. To relax even further, you can read a book, journal, or make lists for tomorrow. If falling asleep is still a challenge, meditation may be sufficiently relaxing to do the trick. If eight hours is not possible to reach by sleeping through the night, consider an afternoon nap–or two. There are many books available about how to better fall asleep and/or stay asleep that you might read as well as podcasts. For chronic problems, a medical sleep evaluation can determine why this is not an occasional problem. Most people know not to ingest or imbibe caffeine later in the day. However, it is best not to drink much liquid within hours of bedtime. In general, it is always useful to keep the room dark and without stimulation so you can relax into sleep.

ELIMINATING SUGAR

Most people do not realize how destructive sugar is to their body. Essentially sugar is a sweet poison that not only creates blood glucose problems but feeds cancers and candida. The best thing you can do to support the functioning of your brain and your body is to eliminate sugar from your diet. Since sugar is addictive and a hidden ingredient in so many of the foods we love and find satisfying it is hard to eliminate. Especially watch out for sodas, sauces, and pastries as they are loaded with sugars as are most processed foods. It is advised to read the mandated labels. Sugar is often on or near the top of the list of any processed food that satisfies your taste buds. However, if it is one of the top three ingredients, that is an automatic indication to put it back on the shelf. Be aware that too many carbs change to sugar and so can also elevate your blood glucose and do the same damage.

EATING HEALTHY FOOD

Eating organic food is the healthiest and also the most expensive. If you are budget constrained, you might want to buy organic for the most contaminated foods like strawberries, apples, spinach, and tomatoes that are subject to more pesticides than others. Always carefully wash and prepare all foods and cut off the skins if possible. Above all, avoid all fast or processed food. While these products taste good, they are not good for you because they contain many ingredients, most unpronounceable, that are unhealthy. Because they contain so many ingredients to be avoided like hydrogenated fats and oils, avoid items with ingredients you cannot pronounce. In general, it is best to avoid the middle aisles of any grocery store or supermarket. All the fresh foods are located around the edges. Your local library has many books full of good advice and good recipes.

COMMUNITY/PURPOSE/SOCIALIZING

The most self-sustaining and supportive activities you can pursue are those that provide meaning and opportunities to be with other people. Aim for interactions with others on a daily basis even if it is only having a phone conversation with a friend or a friendly chat with a grocery clerk or someone else you cross paths with during the day. Participating in community groups or attending church or synagogue programs offer a chance for friendly engagement. There is often more to what is available than religious services, including volunteer opportunities.

KEEP MOVING AND GETTING OUTSIDE

If at all possible, go outdoors on a daily basis, preferably on a walk, which enhances all benefits. However, if desk bound it is crucial to stand up and take mini movement breaks every 15 minutes. If you have a trampoline or an exercise bike at home use it. Clinical studies have indicated seniors who are not sedentary enjoy increased cognitive ability over sedentary peers. Therefore, just get out of your chair and walk around at home if that is all you can do.

It is even better to walk in fresh air so get outside on a regular basis if you can. Look for beauty in wildflowers, cloud formations, and sunsets. If possible, go near a body of water. In San Francisco where I live there are many lakes and smaller bodies of water within my extended neighborhood. And the ocean is only a few miles from my house. No longer is 10,000 steps the suggested amount for longevity benefits. Now doctors advise even 4,000 steps, less than two miles can strengthen your muscles and make a difference in your sense of well-being. The more you move, the less stiff you will feel and the stronger you get.

Even if you have limited mobility and need a wheelchair or other assistance, it is still beneficial to get outdoors. And it is still possible to do more limited prescribed exercises. Sometimes, when you combine walking with window shopping or exploring a new neighborhood, it is easier to go farther. Should you want travel to be in your future, building your leg strength and preserving your mobility is essential. Moving your limbs literally gets the juices flowing. You not only increase the mobility of your joints with every step you take but you are building muscle strength as well. You need to use it to not lose it.

SELF-CARE

Remember to take care of yourself. Too often those who care for others, especially women, leave themselves off their own list. Consider the many ways you can treat yourself to a restorative experience. For me, it is a hot bath with lots of bubbles. Every time I get in a delicious tub, I wonder why I didn't do this more often. What is it you would find most nurturing? Perhaps you will find massages, manicures, and pedicures to be real treats and very effective in the relaxation process. Remember it is also self-care to be kinder in your inner conversations with yourself. Not expecting as much of yourself or berating yourself for anything you did or did not do recently or in the past helps sustain a positive mood.

When younger, I was always in a rush to do more, to be accomplished, achieving something meaningful. At some point, I learned to give myself a break, to slow down and be more present. I allowed myself more time to read, which was always relaxing. Remind yourself you are doing the very best you can and always add into your schedule something that makes you feel better.

MAKING A DIFFERENCE IN THE LIFE OF ANOTHER

Taking care of others and being of service to those in need not only helps them but has the added benefits of diverting your attention from your own debilitating concerns. You will be amazed how little it takes to make a difference in the world and in the life of another person. Even a smile to random strangers can create lifelong memories. I can testify to that from my own experience. I still remember, and am warmed by, the beatific smile of a random stranger I passed on the street decades ago. If you are unable to volunteer at a school, a homeless shelter, or a food kitchen there are things you can do from home, such as participating in hot lines, telephone banks or letter writing campaigns. If interested, check your local volunteer agency for opportunities.

Personal Reflections

What childhood influences most impact you now?

Who were your models? How did they behave?

What kind of situations bring on feelings of Oy?

How do your Oys express themselves in your behavior?

How susceptible are you to taking things personally?

What sort of incidents, situations of circumstances push your buttons?

How do you tend to react?

What can you do to prevent or eliminate such incidents from happening or from triggering you?

How might you respond in a more thoughtful self-nurturing manner?

How might you better prepare yourself to deal with difficult situations by building up your overall sense of well-being?

CHAPTER 5

PURSUING THE PATH OF JOY

"Joy is not a feeling, it is an outlook."
– David Brooks

"Joy is the simplest form of gratitude."
– Karl Barth

Growing up with a father who was depressed and a mother who was always angry, whether she expressed it directly or not, I was taught to be judgmental and fearful. I learned to see the very worst in everything and to be unforgiving. Looking back, this experience of personal childhood trauma may have been my biggest gift since it set me on a life-long spiritual journey. It also gave me my mission to bring emotional support to hundreds of thousands of traumatized children around the world.

I became a social worker to help others as I had wished I could have been helped. I longed for my parents to treat me with more kindness and to want to meet my needs. Unfortunately, that never happened. My life work became a source of emotional support and solace for children living in difficult circumstances. I formed two non-profits. One, called Parents Place, was designed as a family resource center for parents wanting to learn how to become better parents. The other, Caring For Children, described earlier was formed to address the emotional needs of children without parents or children with parents who were unable to take proper care of them. Over a period of 36 years, by inspiring others to pursue the same programs, we eventually reached more than 200,000 youngsters with emotional support and a sense that someone cared. Without my own childhood trauma, I never would have been motivated to pursue such a path. My own trauma gave purpose to my life to trans-mute an Oy into a Joy for youngsters who had so little, and my work more than compensated for the pain of my childhood.

After years of study and years of practice, having acquired considerable spiritual knowledge, I wrote *Climbing the Sacred Ladder: Your Path to Love, Joy, Peace, and Purpose.* The definition I used for joy in that book was "existential delight" and "the expression of an ebullient spirit free from negativity." It still rings true and bears repeating. Joy is our birthright, the fundamental state of our very existence. We need to be vigilant so as not to allow life experiences to deflate our "heightened emotional state." One hallmark of spiritual mastery is to remain joyous even when life breaks your heart. Even when being challenged to your core, like

Scarlett O'Hara, you can remain optimistic and declare, "Tomorrow will be a better day."

Joy is a choice you make regardless of the circumstances of your life. As we have seen, it is easy to be negative, bitter, complaining, and angry. The real spiritual challenge is to get up after being knocked down repeatedly, dust yourself off, and keep on keeping on. It is a frame of mind that looks for the opportunities for Joy that constantly present themselves. It is up to you to open your eyes and grasp them even when they are not so readily apparent. One of the more compelling stories illustrating this principal is of a Buddhist monk being chased by a man-eating tiger to the edge of a cliff. With the tiger in pursuit, the monk lowers himself down the side of the cliff that immediately begins to crumble under his weight. As he is about to fall the monk notices a lone, large, luscious strawberry, growing in a crevice. With the tiger relentlessly approaching, he calmly reaches for it, and puts it in his mouth to savor the luscious flavor.

You too can find moments of joy even in the midst of the darkest days if you learn to pivot from that which depletes your sense of well-being to that which enhances it. Developing a habit of gratitude opens you to conscious appreciation of all the good in your life. Even if all that might be available for you is to appreciate a sunny day, focus on that. This practice will sustain you through the worst of times. Every morning I set the intention for the day, outlining what I want to accomplish and then I fill a journal page of things for which I am grateful. You will be surprised how many there are in your life to be grateful for when you begin to look for them and then pause to appreciate them. You can be filled with joy from something as small as a simmering beautiful beam of light on a wall or a colorful flower growing through a crack in the sidewalk. It can be as significant as having excellent complete coverage health insurance or as seemingly superficial as finding a much-needed parking space when late for a meeting.

The more you experience joy, and the more you celebrate life, the more you will find opportunities to be joyous. What a wonderful merry-go-round to be on.

Since your thoughts determine your focus, and your focus determines the quality of your experience, you can either choose to celebrate this wonderful, beautiful, interesting world or lament that it is difficult, dysfunctional, and disheartening. Would it then not make sense to monitor your thinking and stay focused on what you want to have more of rather than on what you do not want at all?

One of the topics it is best to ignore is society's negative attitude towards the elderly who are denigrated and seen as disposable, irrelevant, and incapable. Do not buy into this way of thinking, which is simply not true. You absolutely can create a happier, more fulfilling, and productive life at any age. It is never too late to create a better tomorrow. Remember back in the 1960s when the dividing line between being young, old, or over the hill was age 40? Now the mantra is you are only as old as you feel. Feeling younger than your chronological age is dependent on preserving your enthusiasm for life and being open to new experiences. Often, out of fear, we cling to what is familiar and seemingly safe. If you are afraid of starting something new that could open a future of possibilities and opportunities, follow the advice of C.S. Lewis who believed, "You are never too old to set another goal or dream a new dream."

SOME PATHS TO JOY

Being open to life requires a spaciousness in your mind, your home, your environment, and your schedule so that there is room for something new to emerge. To create that space requires curating the past clutter in your mind, your activities, your attachments, and your contact list.

Here are some tips to make room for new beginnings inspired by Stephanie Bennet Vogt, author of *A Year to Clear.*

SLOW DOWN

The very first step to upgrading your life is to subdue the internal pressure to do more and more. It is essential that you slow down enough to be more present to your life in this very moment. This advice to slow down when you have become accustomed to rushing, takes effort and repeated practice, but it is essential to improving your quality of life. My daughter, then age ten, tried to teach me to not do "one more thing" by gifting me a precious handmade 'How To' book she created. In addition to teaching me to more correctly assess how long something would take, she listed all the things not to do that would make me late to an appointment. This list included practical tips such as not answering the phone if it rings while you are exiting the house. Sadly, my self-worth was tied up with how much I could accomplish, and I could not follow her sage advice. One day decades ago I was so proud to have crossed 16 tasks off my to-do list. Even though I would not have the energy to do that now, it took a pandemic to stop me in my tracks. Only when forced to stay put by the quarantine restrictions and the many closures was I forced to cease and desist from following my previous standard practice. Since the swimming pool and gym were closed, I had to find alternative ways to exercise at home. Luckily, my gym put most of their classes on Zoom and I got to appreciate not having to drive somewhere to exercise. Eventually, I came to appreciate the beauty of NOT doing. Now, I enjoy a slower paced life, and in some ways, I am even more productive. If I can, you can.

SIMPLIFY

Keeping things simple is good advice at any time in life. This especially resonates in your later years when you have less energy and less bandwidth to deal with life's demands. It is a natural time to simplify your life and let go of possessions no longer wanted, needed, or enjoyed. Dispose of all the clothing you'll never wear again because it does not fit, in more ways than one. You are no longer the same person who acquired them. Others can appreciate them now and you can contribute to their lives by your donation. The same is also true for the books you will never read and other items that may have had meaning at one time, but no longer do.

At the start of the pandemic, I decided to shed at least weekly one brown grocery bag full of no longer relevant possessions and did so throughout the two subsequent years. I am still amazed at what I have let go and don't miss, and even more amazed at the excessive number of possessions that still remain after all I have donated for recycling, donations, or gifts. I am so happy to be seeing surfaces and having more room in my closets and on my bookshelves.

SURRENDER

The best way to surrender to the flow of the present moment with all its beauty is to release all attachments, expectations, desires, and intentions. This does not mean do not have them. It means living with an open hand and watching how the wind blows, to mix metaphors. One thing for sure the pandemic taught was there is absolutely nothing under our control. So, relax into the current moment without worry of the future that is yet to come. This moment is your current reality. Once you release your attachment to a particular outcome and stop resisting the result at hand, you can finally relax and better respond to reality as it is. It does not serve you to insist on a different outcome however more preferable it might be. Any other attitude only leads to disappointment so why not accept what is as it is? That is the path to joy.

SELF-CARE

Nurturing your soul's hopes and heart's desires are as much a part of self-care as pampering your body. Take time also to feed your soul spiritual nourishment in the form of giving and receiving kindness, compassion and caring with like-minded people, by doing things you enjoy and pampering your body with hot baths, massages, and good food.

MAINTAIN A SENSE OF HUMOR AND PERSPECTIVE

While not easy to find a light side to a situation you experience as dark and difficult, sometimes it just helps to lighten up and laugh regardless of the circumstances. Life happens and it is often not easy. Whether you have broken your wrist, or your car has developed serious engine problems, and you really feel like crying, try finding something positive. You can now focus on how you are free of kitchen duty or are unlikely to be injured in a car accident. When your perception of the problem allows for a lighter point of view, you are in the process of developing soul strength.

Just recently, I came home to find my office so full of smoke the air was white. Afraid of a fire, I called the fire department. Five huge firemen arrived and could not find the source. They started emptying the room of all the heavy furniture and all the closet of heavy coats. They even talked about knocking down a wall. I was so astounded that I started to laugh. After more than an hour, they found the cause. It was a magnifying glass on my desk that on an overcast day ignited a fire. It was so absurd I laughed even more.

MAKE LEMONADE

Life has its way of throwing us lemons. When that happens, look for ways that good can come out of an unwanted and unexpected situation with the belief that ALL things are for the good even when there is no evidence for it at the time. It may take years to realize that what you once thought was a disaster was really a blessing. For example, an expensive car accident I recently had led me to a new physical therapist and through him I met others who opened doors to important new opportunities that changed my life in unexpected ways.

Personal Reflections

How do you create joy in your life?

What prevents you from allowing yourself to create or accept more joy in your life?

What are you missing in your life that you would like to have?

What internal constraints do you feel that hold you back?

How can you begin to move beyond these constraints?

What can you do to create even more joy?

What can you do to lighten up and laugh more?

What do you need to let go of that interferes with your feeling more joy?

Who in your life lifts you up or lets you down?

What have you been putting off that would bring you more joy?

What can you do to stop postponing experiences of your joy?

CHAPTER 6
PHYSICAL SELF-CARE

"Self-care is never a selfish act. It is simply good stewardship of the only gift I have I was put on Earth to offer others."
– Parker Palmer

In my salad days, when I was 28 years old living in Manhattan, I would run to catch the subway train even though I knew there would be another one in less than five minutes. At 40, I was still walking the hills of San Francisco in high heels. At 50, I began noticing loss of function when doing yoga. It was upsetting not to be able to stretch as far as I once had. Most frustrating was not having the ability to have my hands touch behind my back in the same way as when I was decades younger. First, it was hard for my hands to meet. Now, not only can I not touch my hands, I can hardly bend my elbows. Initially, I was upset about what I could no longer do; now I appreciate all that I still can. I regularly thank my body for still taking me where I want to go after all these many years. And I realize this is part of the flow of life we all experience. As Leonard Cohen once noted, "My body now aches in places it used to play."

Luckily for me, I always looked and felt considerably younger than my years, even now. Then came the pandemic. For me, as for so many, the world changed. The quarantine disrupted my regular routine, which included many exercise classes and almost daily swimming. My pattern of always being on the go evaporated. There was nowhere to go. My body missed the exercise and responded with weight gain and diminished energy. The change was very hard on me, as it was for millions of others. Within three years, I had gained 15 pounds. I felt as if I had aged at least ten years.

I had to totally shift gears in order to appreciate the space and opportunity for retreat and contemplation created by the shutdown. Having always been spiritually inclined, once I got over the shock of everything being shuttered, I was able eventually to relax into the new reality. Going inward combined with the circumstances and my age led to the origin of this book, which became the silver lining in the lotus pond, to mix metaphors. In the light of the new reality, I had an opportunity to redefine who I was now.

I needed to discover new goals and redefine my purpose to be more in alignment with the new me. It was a gradual transition that led me to writing this book. In retrospect, it was clearly time to let go of what was becoming an increasingly impossible way of life. Ironically, I was experiencing in technicolor what Jung cited as the need to release the impossible dream. Ultimately, I realized I was fortunate to be forced to relinquish my mission because it opened space to discover another purpose more in fitting with my current age and energy. The acceptance of letting go of goals that cannot be achieved stopped me from draining my energy and sense of well-being on the path to futility. Having reached this stage of life, you are offered the same opportunity to redefine yourself in support of evolving your individuality. As you reduce the power of your ego and strengthen your soul, you are able to build new ways of releasing what holds you back and free up energy for emerging new pursuits.

How you see yourself in terms of aging is crucial to how you will conduct yourself as you get older. It is all too easy to limit yourself unnecessarily. You are not your chronological age. My aunt, in her late 90s, refused to share her age even with her doctors. She said my age is a number and it is unlisted.

In addition to a chronological age, your body also has a biological age and a psychological age, the age you feel you are. I am 85 by the measurement of time, under 80 in terms of my body's health and resourcefulness while feeling 28 in my outlook on life. This fits the concept of age-fluidity. Since in truth you are only as old as you feel, you will feel better when you are not identified with a static number of a particular age. Be like Martha Stewart, who at age 80, looked exquisite posing in a sexy swimsuit for *Sports Illustrated*.

My own energy vacillates. Some days I am full of energy and other days can hardly move. I have also noticed that with deep tissue massage I can feel decades younger in less than two hours. Aging is an experience that requires us to be alert to stress and other variables that can diminish our functioning. We can then take action to counteract them. Therefore, avail yourself of the products, services, and experiences that support your feeling and being your youngest self.

The range of physical function may vary considerably. One person can suffer a debilitating stroke at 75, while others are going strong at 90. For Celine Dion, this period began after a serious illness when she was only in her early fifties. Even when you or a loved one cannot continue to live life at the same level because of illness or disability, there is much that can be done to support functioning at a higher level. You begin to feel vulnerable and awaken to your own mortality when you watch your contemporaries begin to decline. For me, it came in my early 80s during the pandemic which, like for everyone else, totally altered my life. Restricting my activities was both a blessing and a curse. I was forced to slow down and deal with the anxiety of a wildly uncertain future. Until then, I had been charging forth full steam ahead, never accomplishing as much as I wanted and then amplifying my efforts to do even more. It was exhausting. Then came the lockdown and the cessation of all interactions, and the activities that had sustained me at a higher level of physical functioning fell away. The frustration of these restrictions caused me to eat more, exercise less, and gain weight.

After I had COVID-19 with its residual fatigue, followed by a hip replacement to restore my ability to move freely without pain, I had no choice but to lean into slowing down and curating my activities. I began to treasure a more moderate pace and now am reveling in one that is even slower.

Part of this process is to gracefully let go of your image of who you once were and what you once could do. We all have memories of what was once executed easily and now is not possible. A friend still full of vitality in his late 70s remembers running track and jumping hurdles in his 20s. His accepting without regret, "I can't do that anymore" is an excellent example for all of us having to face increasing limitations. Eventually there comes a time when it serves to stop remembering what you were able to do once upon a time. You move from the Oy of loss to the Joy of embracing your "new normal" by being grateful for what remains.

At this stage in your life, it is important to focus on building new memories. Taking advantage of experiences and opportunities you are having right now is part of the process that builds the spiritual muscle that compensates for the loss of physical strength. It was this realization that helped me recommit to doing my various practices and to begin writing this book to share with you what I have learned in the hope that what I was learning might be useful in your own eldering process.

Not since adolescence have you had to deal with so many physical changes accompanied by so many mood shifts. In adolescence, your task is to gain new skills; in spiritual aging, it is to relinquish your attachment to many of those skills that have served you well with equanimity. When you stop ruminating about what was and celebrate what remains your life expands. Sheila Malkind, the founder and director of The Legacy Film Festival on Aging happily asserts that despite a recent stroke, "I love to get older with all its challenges. I love to work with those challenges. I look forward to every phase of my life." She is an example to emulate for all of us if we want to live in joy.

Start by loving, honoring, and appreciating your body no matter what. Regardless of the unwanted changes, your body is the foundation on which you build the structure of your life. It is the vehicle through which to express your soul needs in the manifest world. It has given you mobility and independence since birth and will continue to do so for many years to come. Focus on those body parts that are still functioning and pain free. A brief daily body scan helps you recognize and appreciate those parts that are still functional and serving you well. This practice of acknowledgement and appreciation can elevate your experience of the entire day. It can be a part of a daily gratitude practice of appreciating all the beneficial aspects of your life.

Your prime psychological task is to accept your new norm and relinquish what is no longer available without regret. Rather than focusing on what your body once was capable of but can't do any more, focus on the myriad ways your body still functions well. Relax your efforts to swim upstream and go with the flow of what is still to come. Stephen Curry, San Francisco Warriors basketball team superstar, reminds us, "Your body can give out, but your Soul is forever." His words remind us that the real you is not your body.

The ability to function by people the same age can vary wildly. After the age of 55 it takes more work to maintain your level of functioning and feeling of well-being. Even if you can no longer take your body for granted, with more attention and care, you can be functioning effectively for many years to come. Some people are more blessed than others. You will be able to do more when you exercise daily. It is important to be more active when you age. There is great variation that is mostly beyond your control, yet we still must do the best we can. Some can do yoga in their 90s while others have difficulty walking in their 70s. Brava for Margot Fontaine, the ballerina, who danced on stage with Nureyev in her fifties or for me taking ballet lessons in my 80s. And what a fun way to keep my leg muscles strong!

Your health span more than your life span reflects the quality of your life. It takes more than longevity to keep you on the joy side of the equation. Staying active, developing better habits, and learning new skills will preserve your vitality and contribute to your overall health. It is impossible to over-emphasize the importance of maintaining a positive and optimistic outlook. Staying aware of your many remaining abilities is health-inducing while lamenting what was lost lowers your energy, your mood, and can even shorten your life.

For women, loving and accepting yourself despite the cosmetic changes can be the most challenging. At some point, it becomes startling to see your unfamiliar face in the mirror. You have minimal control over the way the passage of time will affect your body. Even when you remain basically healthy unwelcome changes keep arriving. Since the aging process is inevitable and relentless no matter how much it can be slowed down, resistance is ultimately futile. Don't even try. It will depress your spirit, drain your energy, and pocketbook, and not produce the desired results. Rather, celebrate what remains and always remember, a smile disguises many wrinkles.

Ultimately the essence of aging gracefully involves both the full acceptance of the passing of youth and the embracing of the gifts of maturity. Redirecting your focus from the superficial to the essential elements of who you truly are helps you integrate the external changes into your sense of self. Even in this youth-dominated culture it is common to recognize that what really counts is inner beauty.

Reviewing the fundamental spiritual practices explained in Chapter 2 will help you strengthen your soul and, thus, supports your ability to cope with adversity. Additional practices specifically designed to support you in the physical realm follow. Regardless of how many unwelcome changes you are experiencing, there is much you can do to strengthen your body and support your brain. As your thought patterns become more positive, so does your feeling of well-being.

In addition to doing meditation and the other practices previously outlined, now is the time to pay attention to yourself and learn to stay alert to your body's signals and sensations in present time.

The following practices will enhance your well-being in the physical dimension:

ACCOMMODATE YOUR SURROUNDINGS TO YOUR NEW REALITY

It is time to review the setup of your living space and consider changing your environment to be more user friendly. One example is moving items used more often to lower shelves for easier access. I don't know why it took me more than 20 years to realize my coffee cups, which I use frequently, should be on a lower shelf.

Another adaptation is to avail yourself of audio books or videos when reading becomes more difficult. Installing grab bars in your tub and securing your carpets so they don't slip will prevent you from slipping as well. Do all the necessary things to avoid falls. You may want to buy some attractive flat shoes that are less hazardous than wearing higher heels if your balance is compromised. I learned this the hard way when wearing my prettier shoes rather than the ones with rubber soles that would have saved me from a bad fall. Never again. All these adaptations reflect a shift in your orientation to the world. Where you once pushed yourself to adapt to the world, you now realize you can relax and let the world come to you.

STAYING HYDRATED

Drinking sufficient water has long been emphasized to avoid dehydration, which can lead to headaches, brain fog, and irritability among other symptoms. I just learned that dehydration impacts tinnitus and other physical areas of discomfort. So, drink up! And don't limit yourself to eight glasses of water daily. This remains one of the most basic, easiest, and least expensive practices to benefit your body. Drinking filtered water is advised to avoid the unhealthy effects of toxic chemicals that can also create serious health hazards. So be sure to drink sufficient water throughout the day even if you would rather not. Consider buying bottled water in order to eliminate the many chemicals, bad for your health, which are in tap water. You can also boil that water before using it. The healthiest but more expensive alternative is to buy a filter for your faucet.

A simple way to stay on track is to pour yourself eight glasses of water in the morning and make sure you have consumed them all by the end of the day. Tea and coffee do not count as they do not contribute to your being hydrated and can do quite the opposite.

EATING WELL

Beyond eliminating fast foods, junk foods, and processed foods from your diet be sure to consider what additional nutrients your body might need to function optimally. Unfortunately, depleted soils, increased use of toxic chemicals, and corporate farming practices have diminished the nutritional quality of the foods we eat even in our lifetime.

Whenever possible, it is necessary to take restorative supplements to replace the nutrients missing from our food. When possible, for better quality food, buy organic, especially those fruits and vegetables that are most toxic such as strawberries and cucumbers.

GRACEFUL EATING

In addition to eating only healthy, nutrient-dense food to nourish your body and eliminating fast foods, processed foods, and other junk foods from your diet, there lie the questions of how to prepare a peaceful place to nurture. yourself around mealtime. Once you have decided your schedule and prepare your meals, what preparations do you make so that the experience is nurturing of both body and soul? Do you take your time to set an attractive setting in which to serve the food? Do you arrange to eat when not rushed or stressed?

Beyond taking nutrients, avoiding empty calories, and buying organic produce, the whole question is how to structure, plan, and prepare meals in a manner that nourishes your soul as well. How often are meals relaxed despite the busy day? Since you do not live by bread alone, this is the area to develop the other aspects of being present in the experience of eating for pleasure and for health. This is a call to add more consciousness to this aspect of your life so that you relax more and eat less.

MOVEMENT MOMENTUM

An older body needs to keep moving in order for joints to remain well lubricated and muscles stretched and strong. The more you move, the better it is for your body. Strive for 30 minutes daily but even 10 or 15 minutes should give you benefits almost immediately. Recommended exercises include mild aerobic exercise and weightlifting according to capacity. tai chi, qigong, and yoga all use gentle flowing movements that also benefit balance. These practices promote circulation and provide a pleasant routine that will keep your muscles stretched and supple. Strength training, even with small weights or cans of vegetables will help you build, or at least maintain, muscle strength, which otherwise will continue to decrease over time. It is important to include cardio to the point where you are moving vigorously enough to raise your heartbeat. If you have a Medicare Supplement plan, membership at the YMCA, Silver Sneakers senior classes or Zoom classes may be available to you at no extra cost.

SUFFICIENT SLEEP

Sleep is fundamentally important at all stages of life but especially as you age. With aging, sleep becomes interrupted once or twice during the night even if only for a bathroom break. Try to go back to sleep as soon as possible so you can be sufficiently rested. Sleep is restorative to our bodies and is the time when most toxins are eliminated. You need at least eight hours and preferably more to give your body sufficient time to heal. If you get less than that during the night, consider a nap during the day. Sometimes, and I have been experiencing this lately, you may even need a morning and an afternoon nap. Sometimes what seems like excessive sleep is your body's attempt to stave off an infection or other illness. Therefore, respect your body's messages even if what you are experiencing does not follow the model in your mind. If you feel sleepy during the day, it is a signal your body needs more rest, and you should listen to your body. If you have trouble falling asleep or staying asleep, it may be a sign that you are nutrient deficient. Since lack of sleep is one of the man factors that influences memory loss, surely, this is something you want to pay attention to immediately.

MASSAGE, BODY WORK, AND OTHER SUPPORTIVE TREATMENTS

You will be surprised how much younger and more flexible you can feel as a result of body work. One of the worst assumptions as you age is assuming all your discomfort is an inevitable consequence of growing older. Not the case. Much of what you feel has nothing to do with how old you are. Not all aches and pains are due to aging. Some are due to stress, the impact of gravity, or misalignment. If possible, schedule yourself for a relaxing massage that soothes tense muscles, relaxes contracted muscles, and releases built-up tension. In addition to the pleasure of the massage itself, you will enjoy feeling more vitality and well-being than you thought was possible.

Some bodywork practices to consider in addition to therapeutic massage, which is targeted to release the stiffest muscles, include:

- Chiropractic adjustments release the tightness around joints to alleviate pain

- Rolfing techniques are designed to stretch and reposition constricted fascia and other soft tissue

- The Alexander Technique focuses on body alignment

- Polarity is about energy balancing

- Acupuncture is an ancient Chinese method that frees stuck energy that is then available for healing

These modalities contribute to your maintaining a feeling of youthfulness and increased energy.

Personal Reflections

What are you doing now to support your physical well-being?

What more can you be doing in terms of life choices?

What can you stop doing?

What resources do you need to ramp up your self-care?

Who can help support your efforts for self-care?

What are your energy drains?

How can you plug them?

What can you schedule in your weekly routine that would support your goals?

What exercise do you do regularly?

How would you evaluate your results?

How could you improve your nutrition?

How would you evaluate your physical well-being today compared to earlier in life?

What goals can you set for yourself that you will commit to achieve by a given date?

How would your life be better when you achieve those goals?

Describe what your world would look like and how you would feel when you meet your goals?

CHAPTER 7

EMOTIONAL SELF-CARE

"Aging is not lost youth but a new stage
of opportunity and strength."
– Betty Friedan

Watching the inexorable progress of your own aging is never easy. Your experience of the inevitable and inescapable changes may come progressively or intermittently. You, like everyone else, will lose strength, flexibility, and elasticity over time. While there is little you can do to stop the process, you can slow it down as we have discussed. In addition, by accepting, adjusting, and maintaining a positive attitude, no matter what happens, you will begin to value the gifts that come to replace what has been lost.

While you cannot eliminate the process, you always have a choice in how you can respond to your experience of losing the bloom and beauty of youth. These two following examples provide a window into the ways different values and different levels of consciousness deal with the futility of trying to hold back the tides of time.

Jennifer B, 52, had been a beautiful young woman who turned heads wherever she went. She took great pride in her appearance and much of her self-worth was tied up in the admiration she received from men and women alike. She began to feel old in her forties when her skin started to sag. Since her self-esteem was tied to her looks, as her appearance faded so did her feelings of confidence and self-worth. Since she never developed other aspects of her life and had few interests beyond social interactions, there were few ways she could compensate as she got older for the cosmetic changes. Her distress led her to a state of increasing unhappiness.

Molly T, 64, was an attractive woman with many interests and talents she developed over the years. These activities brought her great satisfaction and also presented many opportunities to make friends and widen her circle of acquaintances. As she noticed the changes aging brought, she began to exercise more and pay more attention to her appearance. Although she upgraded her wardrobe and spent more on beauty treatments she did not rely on her appearance for self-worth.

Building emotional resilience enables you to move to a new stage without clinging to the past. These two examples illustrate the two ways of dealing with the decline of youthfulness. One leads to a state of Oy the other to a state of Joy. Which one would you choose?

Clinging to regrets about the past is a waste of time and energy better applied to creating a new tomorrow. There is nothing that you can do to change the march of time. You can only change yourself and by doing so change your future. Still, I reminisce about roads not taken and need to remind myself to keep facing forward and stay focused on what I want my future to be. Resistance to aging is useless. Only by looking beyond appearance and physical prowess can you experience more emotional satisfaction at this stage of life. Therefore, accepting and adapting to unwelcome changes is the essence of aging gracefully.

If this is your case, there are a variety of emotional-based therapies that can help you move forward. In addition to traditional psychotherapy, newer physiologically based modalities including "tapping," or EFT, which stand for Emotional Freedom Technique. This method postulates that saying affirmations while activating parts of your body corresponding to meridian points can stimulate psychological change. Tapping in a systematic way with your hands, on your forehead, under your eyes and other specified points have the power to change thought patterns and the way your life unfolds. I have experienced it myself. I have always had a pattern of police officers stopping me when driving. Sometimes, but not always, they would give me a ticket. Once I did the tapping exercise on my feelings of being bad and deserving of punishment, I had a breakthrough in reframing that thought leaving me in tears. Although many years have passed by now, I haven't been stopped by a police officer again. Another technique known as EMDR (Eye Movement Desensitization and Reprocessing) involves rapid eye movement done with a therapist who reprograms your thoughts while you quickly move your eyes from side to side. These rapid eye movement therapies have proven to be extremely effective with reducing the imprint of traumatic events even with returning veterans marred by their war experiences.

Chip Conley, founder of The Modern Eldering Academy, explains, "We diminish in all kinds of physical ways but that is when resilience and adaptability kick in—when we realize our gifts are no longer physical but emotional, philosophical, and spiritual." Adapting to change and moving on with your life requires releasing psychological and emotional overlays that have kept you repressed and not fully expressive. Shedding what no longer supports you creates the conditions for your true self to emerge. As you move into a new stage of your life, you become increasingly cognizant of the impact of your life experiences and are better able to integrate them into who you are becoming. In order to be more fully self-expressed and authentic you need to know yourself. Releasing the weight of past problems, disappointments, and traumas helps you move onto the next chapter of your life. This also requires eliminating what no longer supports how you function and feel. This involves doing the necessary emotional work of releasing outdated cultural conditioning, society stereotypes, and family influences. Only then can you live from your essence rather than from the expectations of others.

Concentrate on creating a new tomorrow today. You cannot change the past, but you can change yourself and by doing so change your future. What was done was done and nothing can alter what came to pass. Facing the future and focusing on what you want to create is the only path to take.

As you do the work of updating your early conditioning, you can begin using some of the techniques in self-discovery outlined earlier. As you start to discover who you are becoming, you can better embrace what supports your progress and help you jettison the rest. Can you begin to open to new opportunities congruent with whom you have grown to be?

GUIDELINES FOR EMOTIONAL GROWTH

- Be patient in doing these practices as you are priming the pump for your future well-being.

- Forgive your errors in judgment, misplaced trust, missed opportunities, and other past experiences you regret. Be kind to yourself and chalk it up to live and learn. We have all trusted the wrong people and/or not taken the opportunities presented to us that might have led to better outcomes.

- Give up all stories—the meaning you may have bestowed could be more negative than the original event. Keep an open mind. You do not know that another choice would have had a better outcome. Let it go and accept where you are now in your life and what opportunities you have for what might be next.

- Appreciate lucky breaks, dodged bullets, serendipity, synchronicity, and good karma. Keep an open heart. It is important not to misunderstand or misinterpret what was said.

- Curate your memories and preserve the best to draw upon for support and comfort going forward. Having anchors or good memories to refer to when under stress or in distress can shift your mind and, thus, your mood. Remember moments of great kindness, great beauty or great pleasure when feeling alone, unsupported, anxious or unhappy and you can turn your mind from Oy to Joy.

- Accept reality, however painful, especially if you have lost a partner. Seek the support of a therapist or a support group of people who have experienced a similar loss. It helps not to isolate or be alone with unhappy feelings as they tend to escalate when not counterbalanced. Keep bolstering yourself with good memories to buffer the difficult ones.

- Give yourself credit for all you have endured, survived, and learned. Your journey through life is never easy. It takes strength and determination to keep persevering under difficult circumstances often without sufficient support. Sometimes we have to pull ourselves up by our own emotional bootstraps. Give yourself credit for having dealt with what you did as well as you did. You are stronger and more capable than you realize. Own your strength even if it feels unfamiliar or uncomfortable.

- Practice being present and positive in every moment. It is easy to succumb to the woes of the world and let them impact how you feel. By protecting yourself from negativity, you can move forward in an appropriate way based on your best options.

- You can build up your emotional bank account by making regular deposits of positive experiences and feelings. Just as you need a fiduciary savings account in a banking institution, you need an emotional bank account in your heart. Fill it with happy memories and good times so you can dip into it when life is challenging, and emotional reserves are low. You need an emotional buffer to sustain you through hard times and an emotional bank account with stored positive experiences to withdraw when needed. This will happen sooner or later over time, so keep replenishing your emotional bank account so that it doesn't become empty when you make withdrawals.

- Another way to sustain your mood, your sense of well-being and the experience of joy is to do something each day to sustain your good feelings. At least once a week take time for yourself to experience the pleasure of something that stimulates your sense of joy. My favorite activity is visiting a museum and seeing the art. I recently went to an outstanding exhibit of contemporary art that was dynamic and colorful and has stayed with me when clouds are grey.

- Seeking out and creating opportunities for interactive activities can stimulate your mind and satisfy your need for social contact, giving you a much-needed support network.

- Helping another requires taking your attention off yourself, your needs, and your problems in order to shift your attention to another. This is an important diversion when you are not feeling optimal. By not focusing on your own concerns, fears, and upsets you are able to maintain a better state of mind. By helping to make a difference in others' lives, you will make a difference in yours as well.

- Having a hobby to turn to when you are feeling down is a wonderful resource that enables you to better manage your emotions. Hobbies stimulate your mind and divert your thoughts to something more uplifting. They also enhance your skill levels, promote feelings of accomplishment, and provide avenues to connect with others with whom you share a common interest. Getting absorbed in an activity that provides a diversion and a source of social contact elevates your sense of joy. My favorite is playing ping-pong, a skill I developed in adolescence that combines physical activity and social interaction. Each time I play I experience an elevated mood and an experience of well-being.

- Surround yourself with objects that make you smile on the inside. By filling your environment with things that make you smile on the inside, they make you more likely to do so on the outside as well. For me plants, crystals, and colorful mineral stones provide a sense of joy. What fills your heart and enhances your emotional equilibrium?

- Put yourself at the very top of your own list. Don't neglect or deplete yourself by taking care of everyone else and ignoring your own needs. Just as in an airplane where you are admonished to put on your own oxygen mask before trying to help someone else, it is even more essential in daily life to take care of your own needs first so you will be able to meet the needs of others. How else can you be available to care for someone who needs you? I was shocked to discover decades ago when taking a personal development workshop that when it came time to list the priorities in my life, my needs were not even on the list. It was a wake-up call. Women, especially of our generation, have been acculturated as caregivers and often neglect ourselves while taking excellent care of others. It is essential we learn to put ourselves on our own list without feeling guilty.

- Give yourself a time out each day to pause and recalibrate. The very act of sitting, clearing and calming your busy mind, settling your thoughts and emotions is powerful. A religious order I sometimes attend has a practice of having a bell ring several times a day when it is time to just stop, pause, breathe, reset, and return to what you were doing.

Consider which of these practices and options can provide you with the most emotional stability and then seek to enhance that aspect of your life so you can be calm and deal with life's inevitable challenges with equanimity based on restored inner resources.

Personal Reflections

What is your repertoire of "feel good" activities?

Which ones do you utilize and when?

What would make it easier for you to do those activities more often?

What interferes with that happening?

What strategies can you add to raise your spirits when feeling down?

What people in your life are available to support you when needed?

What people in your life make things more difficult for you?

What can you do to avoid or eliminate them from your life?

What other resources can you add to make your life more emotionally satisfying?

CHAPTER 8
MENTAL SELF-CARE

"Thinking is the soul talking with itself."
– **Plato**

Maintaining a healthy mind is paramount to all aspects of healthy aging. It is impossible to feel joy when dealing with cognitive impairment and confusion. It requires clear thinking to navigate life's difficulties and make the appropriate choices and decisions that bring you joy and the peace of mind needed for a happy life.

The meaning you give to the demanding dimensions of your life depends on whether you consider life's difficulties to be frustrating obstacles or as challenges to be overcome. Your experience is in your own hands, metaphorically, and of course, in your mind. An archetypal story is of twins who came across a huge, foul smelling, pile of manure. One twin was disgusted and complaining about the smell, while the other twin was ecstatic. The annoyed twin asked the other, "How can you be so overjoyed?" The other answered with excitement, "With such a big pile of poop, the pony can't be far away."

Which twin are you? And are you willing and able to examine your thoughts and analyze the patterns that form your perceptions? The more you harvest and understand your past, the more you will be able to create a better future. As you increase your understanding of how your thoughts have influenced your important life choices, your greater awareness of how your thought patterns have impacted you means more control over them in the future. The more you eradicate past programming, the more you are free to create a vital, viable future.

That your thoughts create your reality is not a new concept. Doesn't it, therefore, behoove you to think you can, especially if that attitude will bring you more success than if you think you can't? To do so, however, you will need to eliminate the "Dreadful Ds" outlined in the beginning of this book that clutter your mind and keep you stuck. That is your first step towards initiating a new pattern of perceiving and responding differently to life's circumstances with all its dips, diversions, and difficulties. Since like any journey, there will be ups and downs, you will need to proceed with persistence, patience, and faith until the evidence you are on track begins to appear. You are as resilient or as resistant as you allow yourself to be. You choose.

Now that it can be scientifically explained, in physiological terms, why negative thinking is so fundamentally destructive to mind and body, it is even more important to pay heed to your thoughts. The researchers of the decades long ESCAPE Study (Effects of Stress on Cognitive Aging, Physiology, and Emotion) found, like Dr. Becca Levy of Yale, that the chronic stress or repeated exposures to stressors and regular engagement with URTs (unregulated repetitive thoughts) produces chemical reactions that are destructive to your brain. In medical jargon, they predict a "dysregulated hypothalamic-pituitary-adrenal axis function and inflammation… (which) over time will lead to cognitive decline" as well as other physiological indicators of compromised well-being. That study confirmed the conclusion that having persistent, repetitive negative thoughts will damage your brain and your body.

Dr. Daniel Amen, a psychiatrist and neurological expert, also emphasizes the need to eliminate what he calls "Automatic Negative Thinking" or ANTS. According to Dr. Amen the ANTS include the following patterns:

- **ALL OR NOTHING? BLACK OR WHITE—** Thinking everything is either all good or all bad, without recognizing the gradations of many shades of grey in between.

- **GLOBAL THINKING**—Using collective words like always, never, everyone, every time, etc., instead of differentiating circumstances and conditions.

- **FOCUS ON THE NEGATIVE**—Seeing only the worst parts of a situation despite the many positives.

- **UNEXAMINED THOUGHTS AND FEELINGS**—Never analyzing whether the feeling state that impacts the thought is accurate.

- **GUILT BEATING**—Using words like should, must, and ought, which invoke excessive guilt.

- **LABELING**—Describing yourself or others with negative names like "loser." Summing up a situation or a person with one word obviously does not do justice to the complexity of life.

- **FORTUNE TELLING**—Predicting the worst in every situation based on no apparent evidence.

- **MIND READING**—Thinking you know what someone is thinking without checking it out for accuracy.

- **BLAME**—Projecting onto someone else something that you feel guilty about but do not want to admit, even to yourself. This thinking limits your ability to accurately appraise a situation or person.

- **JUMPING TO CONCLUSIONS**—Making an assessment without examining the evidence or investigating points of view leads to this frequent error in judgment.

- **FUTURIZING**—Making a projection that something will or will not happen when there is no evidence that will be the case is another example of thinking that does not serve you.

- **FANTASIZING**—Allowing one's self to be led astray by daydreams or wishful thinking having no grounds in reality.

- **DENIAL**—Refusal to look at or fully consider all facts in a situation is a result of the person not being able to face a painful conclusion.

- **EXAGGERATING OR MINIMIZING**—Maintaining that the situation under examination is either of greater or lesser concern, danger, value, etc., than justified by objective evaluation of evidence.

- **FILTERING**—Using only a portion of the evidence to make a determination as to the accuracy of your thinking.

Which of these defense mechanisms, as they are called by Anna Freud, do you tend to use? Pay attention going forward to your cognitive patterns that may distort your reality.

Just as you would get an exterminator to eliminate an ant infestation in your house, so do you need to exterminate the mental ANTs that contaminate your mind. Dr. Amen goes on to confirm the results of the ESCAPE study by explaining how uninterrupted, repetitive, negative thoughts lead to anxiety and depression over time. Because those persistent thoughts create chemical changes in your brain that are damaging to your well-being, it is imperative you eliminate them immediately. This is another instance where the practice of meditation will serve you in obtaining clarity, and being more able to manage your thoughts.

SUGGESTIONS FOR INCREASING MENTAL STRENGTH

Mind-Strengthening

Most important is to keep the mind activated in order to maintain brain function. There is no other area of life where use it or lose it is more important and significant. It is crucial to keep exercising your brain with mind games, memorization, and most importantly, learning new skills. It doesn't even matter what you are learning although learning a foreign language is particularly effective because of all the memorization and may even be useful for travel, which also counts as a beneficial new experience. And if it includes movement such as tai chi, zumba or even yoga, so much the better. Anything that interests you will do. Just do it!

It also helps to keep reading on a regular basis. A book club adds the benefits of social interaction and stimulating conversation. It may be both interesting and helpful for you to keep up with your profession like a 92-year-old lawyer who no longer practices but nonetheless takes courses for qualifying for bar certification. So, plan to keep as active mentally as physically. You can do both simultaneously with dancing, which has been proven to be the most effective activity of all and may be the most fun as well.

MENTAL ACCOUNTING

Tracking your thoughts during the day and keeping a record of all negative thoughts for later review will, over a period of time, enable you to determine persistent themes and or repetitive patterns that you can then address.

DEEPER INSIGHTS THROUGH JOURNALING

Starting a journal to write down your thoughts and experiences helps you to go deeper in your increasing ability to access the content of your mind. Make this an experience you would enjoy to ensure you will do it consistently. Choose a journal and pens that are pleasing and trigger feelings of joy. Then structure your environment to make your daily entries easier to sustain. In this way you are supporting yourself for success. Tracing your thoughts so you can see patterns and gain insights gives you the information needed to make the necessary adjustments.

FRIENDS AND SOCIAL CONNECTIONS

Feedback from friends can give you valuable information and insights into attitudes of which you may not be aware. Many years ago, I had a friend who once during a phone conversation told me, "I am tired of hearing you put yourself down. If you can't stop belittling yourself, I don't want to talk to you anymore." Because I valued her friendship enormously, that was enough to shift my behavior. Years later when I thanked her and told her I had stopped that behavior, she replied, "Now, it is time to build yourself up."

AFFIRMATIONS

Until now you have been learning how to eliminate negative thought patterns from your mind. Now it is time, as my friend wisely advised me, to build yourself up. One way to do that is by using affirmations to fertilize your mind. Affirmations are positive thoughts that plant seeds that will nurture new patterns of thoughts and beliefs. An affirmation is usually an "I" statement claiming for yourself in the present moment what is not yet available in reality. A fitting example for this section would be "I release toxic thoughts." Others include, "I choose to see the silver lining in all things" and "Money comes to me in perfect ways from unexpected sources." By repeating and reprograming your mind, if these statements are not yet true, they soon will be.

Whether you repeat them aloud, say them in your mind, or write them down on a daily basis you are training your mind to focus on positive and supportive thoughts and feelings that elevate your experience of life itself in the present moment. Words of self-acceptance, affirmation, praise, or support for yourself and those around you is a circle that supports your sense of well-being and community. Because the better you feel the more likely your thoughts will be positive and life enhancing, this is the opposite of a vicious cycle. Rather it is a spiral up to a greater sense of agency and authenticity.

Affirmations are always positive and often start with the words "I Am" since you want to declare into being what you want to manifest in yourself. Sometimes it is a statement of what you want to manifest in your life. I write affirmations on a regular basis to keep my mind on what I want or what I want to be. I have discovered an app called I AM that provides multiple affirmations to contemplate each day that are more creative and complete than anything I could come up with on my own. Today's affirmations include:

- I enjoy each moment without worrying about what is next.

- I am at peace with who I am now and excited about who I can be.

- I now begin the most loving chapter of my life.

- I know that anything I lose is being replaced by something much better.

In contrast, persistent negative thinking is not only detrimental for your body, as has been described, but it is also dangerous for your soul. Thousands of years ago, Plutarch, an ancient Greek philosopher, wrote that what we think in our mind becomes our outer reality. Pollyanna, a fictional heroine of my childhood who only saw the good in everything including experiences like breaking her leg, which most people would find hard to put a positive spin on, had learned an important secret of life. You too can learn to nurture only positive thoughts opening you up to more opportunities to experience joy.

In time you will begin to become more congruent with your authentic self. You will live more and more in alignment with your desires, your beliefs and your values. Even when you are in a situation beyond your control, you can choose to be positive regardless of the circumstances. It is easy to criticize and be dissatisfied; it takes soul strength to see the best in a less-than-ideal situation. A prime example of this kind of thinking underlying spiritual aging is the story of Sally, an elderly woman moving into assisted living. As she was being shown to her new apartment, staff expressed their hope that she would like her new home and be happy there. Sally replied, "I already like it. I made up my mind in advance that I would be happy here."

As you gain greater control of your habitual ways of thinking, you also gain more understanding from past lessons and, thus, more control over your future. When you relinquish your regrets, dissatisfactions, and the decisions that got you there, you begin to appreciate how enormously fortunate your life has been despite mistakes. Patience and faith will sustain you until the evidence of change becomes apparent.

Researchers investigating brain plasticity, the idea that the brain is not a fixed entity, found the brain is able to develop new neural pathways throughout life. In fact, there are many ways to develop a better brain at any age. While your brain may be healthy, many patterns of thought often are not. Since your mental habits can change, so can you. Remember, this is a journey that continues for the rest of your life.

Personal Reflections

How would you describe the level of mental health in
the home you grew up in?

What did you learn that was useful in terms of
learning how to think about life?

What did you learn that was not useful in terms of
learning how to think about life?

How would you describe your current state of mind?

Are you happy with the state of your mind?

Which of the ANTS do you tend to utilize?
How often?

What actions can you take to dispel them?

Which affirmations, if any, do you find useful?

What would you advise your future self?

List of Affirmations

Make a list of those affirmations that it would be useful for you to repeat throughout the day to remind yourself of the need to change your thoughts or your feelings.

CHAPTER 9

SPIRITUAL SELF-CARE

"When the body begins to decline, it is time to no longer identify with the body but with the consciousness of which it is a vehicle."
– **Joseph Campbell**

In a society that values the externals of life: material possessions, status, power, and wealth, there are few incentives or supports to developing a spiritual life. Yet, your ultimate goal is to live from a spiritual center that gives meaning to who you are and what you do. A sensitive soul in this society on steroids needs protection from the stimulation and stress of daily life. Especially when retired and somewhat shielded from the vast marketplace of our current culture, you can carve out private time for spreading your spiritual wings and soaring to a higher plain of existence.

When more soul conscious, you automatically pay more attention to the voice of your authentic self. You are more in tune with what it wants, needs, and feels. You become more skilled at tapping into the love, joy, peace, and purpose lying dormant below the demands of daily life. By paying attention to your internal interests, instead of external pressures, you begin to live life from the inside out. One of the benefits of aging is to be able to step back from your daily routine and reevaluate your life in order to determine how YOU want to live. This is your opportunity to curate your life and design a way forward that brings you much greater joy.

Use this opportunity to ponder what you would like to add or like to change to make your life more fulfilling. Include how you are scheduling yourself and how you could do more of what would provide greater satisfaction and joy. Despite all your perceived responsibilities and the needs of others in your life, you can take better care of your own spiritual needs. That should be your highest priority.

This week after a lengthy dental appointment and a long list of maintenance items that monopolized my schedule, I made sure to stop at my favorite spot in our local park where pigeons and sea gulls gather near a lake. Watching them compete and cavort at my feet for the grain I had brought to feed them totally lifted my mood. How can you include more of such experiences in your daily life? The more you allow yourself such diversions the happier and more in touch with your soul you will be. You will have a greater sense of how to savor the flavors of what life has to offer. As you create more of such experiences that bring you great satisfaction the more you will experience joy on a regular basis. Whether the chirping of a bird or the aroma of a luscious rose, your goal is to be fully aware of being alive. To have a peaceful spiritual life requires pausing periodically to nourish your inner spark of divine energy.

Who you are and why you are on earth goes far beyond labels, (gender, race, ethnicity, religion), or roles (parent, worker, son or daughter, spouse). That kind of categorizing reduces the depth and richness of your soul. When you do the work as outlined in earlier chapters, you will develop the inner knowing of your true magnificence. Despite a material world that values possessions over people and money over meaning, when you can be fully expressive by realizing your duty is to your higher self, or soul. Releasing the ingrained beliefs, the emotional pain, and the entrenched patterns of behavior, you begin to explore what lies beneath in order to discover who you truly are here and now. When you make time to move beyond the problems of everyday life in order to experience the joy of being alive, you are profoundly expressing spiritual self-care.

Follow these principles of conscious aging and you will be able to develop the core strength, knowledge, insight, resilience to participate in life in a new way, from a new perspective, living your life to the fullest. This becomes increasingly easier as you continue to age and continue to sage.

Here are some of the gifts that come with spiritual aging:

- Taking a longer view of your life.

- Learning there are many perspectives from which to view things.

- Realizing, over time, that what you thought was a disappointment, turned out to be a blessing.

- Recognizing the strength and savvy you have accumulated along the way.

- Appreciating each day as a gift. Some say that is why they call it the present.

Frank Lloyd Wright, who did more than a third of his creative work over the age of 80, revealed that the longer he lived the more beautiful life became for him. You too can become more appreciative of the gift of life and the world around you with increasing age. This is a sign of your increasing spirituality. The more spiritual you become, the less you take for granted. The more you increase your ability to take life as it comes, the more you need to learn to dance with what you cannot escape. While over time you can begin to mold your circumstances, you must first come to terms with a reality you do not like and have no power to change. This is the ultimate lesson of radical acceptance. The secret is not to look back or in the mirror.

In his book, *Ageless Body, Timeless Mind,* Deepak Chopra describes an experiment involving a group of educated 70-year-old male college grads who were isolated at a retreat center for more than a week. They stayed in a controlled time-capsule environment that recreated the year and the culture of their college days in 1959. There were no televisions or contemporary newspapers. Instead, the headlines and the music were from their college era, as was their style of dressing and the topics under discussion.

Extensive physical evaluations with body measurements were taken before and after participating. The results were striking. Not only did the men feel and look younger and gain in mobility, but their biomarkers had changed to those of younger men. Surprisingly even their fingers had lengthened. This confirms previously cited research regarding the importance of developing a youthful mindset to maintain a youthful body. This can be observed in daily life as you often encounter people who look remarkably younger than their chronological age. You too can remain youthful in spirit and your mind, and your body will follow. If they can do it, so can you.

Moving from Oy to Joy is an inside job on your way to greater personal freedom. Doing so is a process of relaxing your ego and extending your sense of personal identity beyond your small self. Doing so entails stripping away the baggage of a lifetime with detachment and integrity. It helps to have a sense of humor so that you do not take everything so seriously. Cultivating a more spiritual life is part of this passage. The natural process of withdrawing energy from the world and repurposing it for introspection and personal development brings us to the work of psychoanalyst Carl Jung, a contemporary of Freud, who also made profound contributions to the understanding of aging. His theory was that aging entails personal and spiritual growth and especially the "gradual spiritualization of consciousness." His thesis was that longevity serves a dual purpose for "the sake of society and the sake of our soul." Even though getting older is mostly seen as something to be dreaded in our age-aversive, youth-oriented culture, Jung reframed it into a vital stage of psychological and spiritual development.

Jung's concept of the spiritualization of consciousness includes:

- Living more in the future than the past
- Having a goal to grow into
- Looking for and finding answers within
- Broadening your outlook
- Saying no to stressors

- Savoring the moment
- Reprioritizing values and desires
- Sacrificing ego goals no longer physically possible
- Learning better forms of self-expression
- Extending the boundaries of your consciousness and self-awareness

Developing these internalized skills is a psycho-social curriculum for elders. As you replace your get up and go with slower but deeper periods of self-introspection and self-expression, you strengthen your ability to live from more authenticity.

Among the tasks of aging are:

- Raising your level of self-awareness and greater consciousness about the world

- Greater acceptance, more equanimity, greater responsiveness and less reactivity

- Reflecting on your life, telling your life story, living by example, and supporting others

- Redefining yourself

- Letting go of aspirations that are not attainable and deplete your sense of well-being

- Nourishing your higher self

As you learned to get go of certain goals, relationships, and cherished dreams, which must be abandoned with grace and liberate yourself exhausting efforts towards unachievable goals, you can begin to devote yourself to pursuing what is possible to the best of your ability.

Your blossoming individuation frees you from ego dominance and strengthens your deepest aspirations. This is essential for your rebirth as an elder.

BASIC GUIDELINES

- Remember, the meaning you give to an experience or an event may not be the whole truth.

- Do a life review (see homework) embracing what you have learned about yourself along your path.

- Accept the reality about how life has changed, especially if you have lost a partner.

- Be adaptable, finding new ways to manage and function.

- Focus on the here and now, who you have become and what is still possible.

PRACTICES ELEVATING YOUR EMOTIONS AND YOUR LIFE

GRATITUDE

Do you ever stop and consider how fortunate you are to be living as peacefully and well as you are on this war-torn planet? With more than 100 million refugees, migrants, displaced, homeless, and food-insecure people with no access to medical care, if you have a roof over your head, a bed to sleep in, food in the refrigerator, and money in the bank you are better off than 95% of people alive today. Every morning when you wake up you may find a good time to make a list of all the things you are grateful for. I fill a page in a small journal every morning when I wake up as it will set the tone for your awareness as you go through your day. Take nothing for granted.

Gratitude is a preferable alternative to the pity party approach. Even when life, with its repeated frustrations and seeming defeats, has depleted you, you can find beauty and support to continue on from the world around you. A friend of mine described her despair after a painful break-up. As she was mourning the loss of a future together, while lying in her bed in the dark, wallowing in her sadness, she made the conscious decision to change her state of mind by focusing on what she was grateful for. As she looked around the room and saw the many possessions that brought her joy, she was able to shift her mood in a flash. This healing power of gratitude was the same experience of another friend recovering from a severe illness that left her immune system so severely compromised she was confined to bed without companionship. Unable to read or even watch TV, she decided to say 100 blessings a day. From her sickbed, she could see beautiful clouds and luscious green grass and the flowers by her bed and that helped her face her challenges with grace and gratitude.

An attitude of gratitude provides the grease to smooth your remaining ride through life. Pollyanna had it right. There is so much to be grateful for in every moment of your life despite difficulties, disagreements, and decisions that didn't work out. Remember, gratitude is an option available at any time.

FORGIVENESS

Forgiveness is the act of letting go of your anger, hurt, and even righteousness regarding some memory or person that continually gives you grief. Even if you have been holding on for far too long, you should realize most likely the object of your upset has moved on. The only person being impacted by the pain, anger, and disappointment is you. Are you familiar with the image of pointing a finger at someone and having three fingers pointed back at you? It is time to stop holding on and move on. Forgive yourself first and then release anything that interferes with a full pardon of the other person regardless of what they have done. It will be a relief to let go of a lifetime of anger, resentment, judging yourself and others. However, forgiveness is not easy, and just when you think you have done so, old feelings and thoughts pop up to show you there is more to do.

Forgiveness also involves releasing any upset, shame, and blame, as well as any expectations that things could have been different from what they were. It means fully accepting and totally letting go of all the memories that make you mad or miserable. And most of all, it means forgiving yourself.

LOVE

Learn to truly love unconditionally with a love that does not waiver with circumstances, changes in appearance, or the vicissitudes of a relationship. However, the primary person you need to love is yourself. Unless you can totally love yourself, you will always doubt the love of the other person. If you can't fully love yourself, how could they? Just as Hamlet cites, "Be true to yourself or else you cannot be true to any man." Also true is the corollary that you need to love yourself, or you cannot love anyone. Love starts with you. Your ability to love is determined in large part by how and how much you were loved as a child. If you were not treasured, enjoyed, played with, taken care of, there is no doubt that your ability to love others is damaged. Your first goal is self-love. Then you can love others.

If you were not fortunate enough to be loved deeply and unconditionally, you can move past your deficit if you do the necessary hard work to correct it. "Love your neighbor as yourself" does not amount to very much if you do not truly love yourself. That is the work of a lifetime. While all that we have covered in the previous pages is basic and vital to your journey through later life, your most valuable trait as an elder is your resistance to letting life get your down. Rather, your motto is "get up and get at it." Your ability to do just that is a reflection of your resilience or your capacity to "bounce back" when you are down. It also includes your ability to envision a better future when the signs for a fruitful outcome are not yet apparent. It means continuing to pursue your goals without any evidence that you will succeed in achieving them. The Resilient Rs are those attributes that repeatedly enable you to move forward in life with a refreshed, reenergized, reinvigorated, renewed and reawakened spirit regardless of circumstances.

THE RESILIENT Rs

These attributes that will carry you forward because they refresh, reenergize, and reawaken your spirit.

REVIEW – Reviewing your past gives you an opportunity to reconsider old interpretations and make a present time division between what was then and what is now. Then you can choose where it serves you best to put your attention on your goal to redesign your life going forward.

REFRAME – Being able to examine the point of view creates space for greater understanding and a broader perspective. This is one of the basic fundamentals for personal growth.

REAFFIRM – When cherished values, interests, activities, relationships, and beliefs are still a good fit, you are reaffirming that you are at peace with who you are and how you want to live your life.

RECHARGE – Self-care and restorative activities that regenerate your energy and enhance your sense of well- being bring a higher level of energy to your activities.

RENEW – Bringing fresh energy to a relationship, an enterprise, a mindset creates opportunities for self-expression that enables you to continually grow into your best self.

REVITALIZE – Staying present and releasing the past opens the way to the future in new and unanticipated ways since you are no longer tethered to what has been holding you back.

RESILIENCE – Being able to bounce back and rebound is an important trait to be cultivated as it is resilience that brings you back to center and restores balance to your life. Like the child's weighted plastic clown, no matter how much life knocks you down, you bounce back up.

Personal Reflections

On a scale of 1-10, indicate your current level of spirituality ?

Who, if anyone, was influential in your spiritual development?

Have you become more spiritual as you age? Describe.

What would support your further spiritual development?

What can you do to reach or maintain that spiritual state?

In what ways do you try to enhance it?

Do you belong to a spiritual community?

If not, what can you do to find one?

Would you be interested in creating one?

How do you fuel your soul with supportive or sustaining activities?

How do you experience life differently when you are in touch with your soul?

What is your experience of life when you are not?

CHAPTER 10

MOVING FORWARD

"Life is no brief candle to me. It is sort of a splendid torch
which I have got hold of for the moment, and I want
to make it burn as brightly as possible before
handing it on to future generations!"
– George Bernard Shaw

As you reach the end of your journey from Oy to Joy, no doubt you have discovered as did Bonnie Prudden, the female fitness guru who was a contemporary of Jack LaLanne that, "It takes a lot of strength to grow old." Even more than physical stamina, soul strength is necessary to creating a future in alignment with your whole self. Wisdom and a sense of purpose provide the resilience crucial to dealing with life's challenges. You have learned to maintain a positive outlook and focus on what can be created or changed without wasting time on those aspects you are powerless to change. Instead, keep your eyes on the prize and strive to do what you can from a place of spiritual serenity. It is in that spirit that Mother Theresa declared, "I will never attend an anti-war rally, but I am happy to attend a peace demonstration."

The older you get, the more you realize that life rarely complies with personal preferences. You learn to release any remaining illusions of personal control because you now know that anything can happen at any time and usually does. Therefore, the motto "Man proposes, God disposes" becomes a mantra as you learn more to accept what comes our way and not to pursue what does not. This is where your "A" Game supports you in developing the soul strength needed to deal with the changes that come with aging.

Your greatest lessons come with the increased challenges that arise when your strength diminishes and time gets shorter. This is your true testing ground. This is where you can practice what you have learned and apply the wisdom you have acquired. You can deal more effectively with life's demands when you are no longer draining energy in resistance to them. As you age and have fewer illusions and more perspective, you are more comfortable with releasing long-held treasured dreams, goals, and ambitions in order to make room for what is still possible. You have learned that letting go of what is not attainable is necessary in order to use your energy for what is. Your job at this time of your life, more than any other, is to "stop trying to push the river" so you can "go with the flow."

This chapter of your life offers a final opportunity to become the person you were born to be. Your task in this last part of your life is to enhance your wisdom and develop your purpose to make the world a better place. It doesn't matter whether you have a major calling or a seemingly insignificant bit part like the unnamed man in the Bible who leads Joseph to find his brothers. Identified only as "man" he never knew how crucial his small part was to the unfolding of the entire biblical story.

Your contribution to the world may be profound or mundane. It may be simply to bring a smile to those who need one. It may be knitting hats for foster children or providing a leadership role to solve a community problem. If you do not already know your purpose, be open to its presenting itself in the form of an opportunity to bring your gift to the world. When you discover where you are needed, it is up to you to follow the prompts.

Many have been able to find that part of themselves in ways not previously dreamt of. Speaking in his old age, Henri Matisse described the infirmities and limitations that required him to develop the new techniques that radically changed his art and added that it had taken him the experience of a lifetime to be able to reach the point that he was capable of doing so. It took all that he experienced before to get to that point. Leonard Cohen wrote his last song at 82 before his death. You too have the opportunity to explore newly discovered parts of your personality waiting for self-expression. There is no end to your ability to adapt in a way that enables you to live in a new way from a new place with new experiences leading you forward to a new outcome in your life.

Jean Shinoda Bolen author of *Goddesses in Everywoman and Gods in Everyman* calls this process of finding your true inner self, the framework for expressing your unique essence, the process of "individuation." And in contemporary terms, Oprah Winfrey sums up our journey to maturity as "with each passing year we become more of the person we were meant to be." Carl Gustav Jung calls this process "the privilege of a lifetime" adding only by living long enough to do the inner work can you "become who you truly are."

You have won the lottery of soul development by virtue of your long life. You have been granted an opportunity to pursue a new path and explore a new way of being in the world. Building on your psychological maturation and the skills acquired over time from various life experiences, you have developed a more profound sense of yourself and how you want to express that self for the rest of your life. Recognizing that you no longer are who you were and not yet who you will be requires your commitment to creating your new you. Take all necessary steps to move full speed ahead without letting the issues of the past block your progress as you create more appropriate behaviors for this stage of your life.

It was this growing ability to face your human imperfections that Maya Angelou referred to when she asserted, "Do the best you can until you know better. When you know better, you can do better." As you release the grip of old patterns from your past, you can open a space for growing new more appropriate ways of dealing with this stage of life. As a young clinician, I worked with a married couple experiencing great discord. The wife had many complaints about the past and the husband was trying his best to get beyond them in order to create a new future without much success. Finally, in exacerbation, he exclaimed, "Put all your angers, grudges, criticisms, disappointments in a big trunk and sit on it." He instinctively knew that focusing on what had repeatedly happened previously would not create the space to take their relationship in a new direction. Repetitive thoughts and reactions only deepen the groove that keeps you stuck. When there isn't much time left, it is imperative to get on with it.

Like the statue hidden in stone, your pure soul is now finally ready to be revealed. Many of your enculturated erroneous ideas and beliefs evaporate. Letting go of previous hallmarks of your identity opens room for new and more appropriate choices that express who you are now. Let go of your old identity so you can update how you see the world. Previously, you defined your life by status, accomplishment, and acquisition rather than by your inner light and the small, still, muffled voice that can now be heard. The true you lay dormant. Now it is time to be reborn.

You do this by staying centered in yourself, present in the moment, and rooted in being rather than doing or having and allow space for your new self to emerge.

This final chapter provides the context for the last chapter of your life. It teaches you to live each day fully unto itself without worry (future) or regrets (past). You have realized there is no value to looking back at what is over and done. You have learned to accept all it entailed without any need for any part of it to be any different. You now realize that you would not be the person who you are now if the past had been different. It took all those experiences to make you who you have become. And if the past had been different, your present would have been different as well with no guarantee it would be any better. So, appreciate the gifts of the present moment and anticipate, with pleasure, a future yet to come. Above all, as you accept yourself as you are, complete with benefits and boo-boos, you can better approach your future from a place of equanimity and joy.

Like fine wine, aging into your fullest essence takes time and cannot be rushed. The errors and other impediments along the way are an intrinsic part of the process. It is not a cliché to say, "The best way to become old and wise is first to be young and foolish." What you experienced in your past was your school for the lessons you needed to learn. Now, having arrived at that later-in-life point, you can treasure what you now know that you didn't know then.

Inevitably with age comes a level of wisdom and under-standing not available earlier. You can now see how all your mistakes and missteps were actually necessary footprints along your path to the present. And you realize that although you are now wiser, you are not actually wise because there is always more to learn. And you learn that what was true for the past may not be true for the future. Like Ulysses who had smooth sailing on his way to Troy, but suffered disaster after disaster on his way home, you might discover that what had worked during the first half of life no longer does in the second. Like Ulysses, you may need to discover or develop new patterns to get you where you want to go.

Wisdom is basic to your clarity of purpose which requires relinquishing illusions and attachment to beliefs, desires, dreams that cannot be realized. As a social worker, having grown into adolescence after the horrors of World War II, my illusion was that the world would be a place of increased humanity fueled by what was learned from the horrors of the recent past. And, as a corollary, if I worked long enough and hard enough, I could midwife the birth of a better world. Instead the world got worse faster than I could ever have imagined. Even though I was increasingly exhausted and saddened by the futility of my efforts, it was excruciating to let go of my mission. Facing facts was enormously painful, but then so was chasing windmills. Reluctantly and painfully, I surrendered my illusions and accepted not only my limitations but, for one reason or another, the reality that humanity was on a very different page.

That moral of such naïve overreaching is echoed in the following story of the traveling preacher determined to change the world. In his zeal, he neglected his family and their economic well-being in his efforts to reach people in faraway places. He would travel great distances for long periods of time. After preaching to large numbers of people, he would return home exhausted with no evidence of perceptible change. The following year, he decided to limit his efforts to his own country and went off again on an extended tour that, again, failed to make the difference he was wanting. So, the next year, he decided to restrict his efforts to his own province and eventually to his own city. Even then, he failed to make a difference, so he decided to focus on changing his own family, which too was a failed effort. Finally, he realized the only person he could change was himself.

Wisdom helps you discern what is doable. You have learned to abandon any illusions of what is not possible and only takes you totally off track. Therefore, to the best of your ability, have an open mind and be willing to take feedback and advice. There is a great deal you can contribute to making the world a better place on the personal level once you limit your goals. Be realistic about what is possible. I always had lofty goals for my clients as a young social worker and my supervisor would repeatedly tell me to limit my goals. You can always create another level once the first ones are accomplished and there is no sense of failure if you do not. Do what you need to do to do the best you can and then be grateful for all you can do.

SOME GUIDING TIPS

- Know that JOY is an inside job. It doesn't come from what does or does not happen around you. It is not circumstances or the behavior of others that determines your ability to be joyous but your attitude and interpretation of them.

- If you must review painful experiences, do so with perspective and detachment. Look to see if there is another side to your perceptions and perspectives that could have a softer landing in your heart.

- Do a daily gratitude practice. Counting your blessings is so easy to do if you only look around the world and realize how fortunate you are.

- Affirming "I am a beloved child of God" instead of "Poor me" allows you to be grateful regardless of circumstances. There is always something to praise that brings you pleasure even if you may need to dig deep.

- Perform a burning bowl ceremony by writing on little pieces of paper what you want gone from your life and then in a ritual, alone or with friends, burn the papers in a bowl in a safe place.

- Write letters to people who have upset or offended you. Empty your heart and fill as many pages as you need to fully empty yourself of upset but DO NOT mail them.

- Express your creativity. The form does not matter, the shift in cognitive activity produces a sense of well-being by diverting your mind from negative thoughts.

- Be vigilant in shifting negative thoughts to positive ones. Take an index card and on one side, list what you appreciate about yourself and on the other side, what you are grateful for in your life and use it as a reminder when you are feeling down and need lifting up.

- Be a source of joy to others. Even a smile and the smallest act of kindness can go a very long way to brighten someone else's day. As a bonus, the goodwill generated comes back to you and uplifts your spirits as well.

- Make time to play. It is crucial you allow yourself to relax and enjoy yourself, to catch up on activities that give you pleasure and develop friendships that will hold you in good stead. The Pickleball craze is a good example of how to get exercise and make friends at the same time.

- Be optimistic–no reason to worry in advance or for no reason about what may never happen.

- Choose doing what makes your heart sing.

- Incorporate activities that make you feel good on a regular basis.

- Avoid doing things or being with people that drag you down.

- Hang out with people who make you feel good; the more the merrier.

- Eliminate sources of negativity starting with the news. What is happening in the world can only make you depressed and impotent since there is NOTHING you can do to make a difference. Use the internet for a quick update without getting absorbed.

Personal Reflections

How did this book resonate with you?

In what ways was it useful?

What would have made it more useful?

Which of the suggestions, strategies, or exercises in this chapter would you follow?

What would you tell your younger self to do what you now understand that you did not know before?

What are you willing to change now that you were not ready to do earlier?

HOW WILL YOU MOVE FORWARD?

"Age has no reality except in the physical world. Our lives are eternal which is to say that our spirits remain as useful and vigorous as when we were in full bloom."
– Gabriel Garcia Marquez

"Even in old age they will bear fruit,
They will remain vital and green."
– Psalm 92

Just as you completed Personal Reflections about your starting point at the beginning of this book, now is the time to complete the following Personal Reflections about how you will use the things you have learned. These are the reflections to take with you as you move forward.

Personal Reflections On Your Plan

How do you want to be as your best self in your remaining years?

What do you need to add or eliminate to enhance your life experience?

What steps do you need to take to move in a new direction?

How comfortable are you about forging your own path without the approval of others?

How do you deal with your fears and concerns about leaving your comfort zone?

What is it you fear? What is the best way to deal with it?

What can you create to support your new
understanding and keep you on track?

What rituals can you create which will support your
maturation as an Elder?

How can you shift your attention to being more
present in the moment?

APPENDIX A
REFLECTING ON YOUR PAST
TO CREATE YOUR FUTURE

Try some of these additional activities:

LIFE REVIEW

As part of your transition to a new phase of your life, it is time to review the path that brought you to where you are now as a guide going forward. Your life review begins by gathering memories of the various events and experiences so you can organize them in a way meaningful to you which can be chronological or not. Reviewing your history provides a chance to develop a new perspective on the events and experiences that have brought you to this point in the long trajectory of your life. The more you devote time and attention to this process, the more you will uncover, and a more cohesive sense of how your life has unfolded to this point will become available to you. You can enrich your memories and your relationships by sharing common experiences and memories with family members and close friends. Perhaps you will even have opportunities to learn more about your family history.

Begin by making a written chronicle of recalled incidents, personalities, and early childhood impressions in any order they come to you.

This written record not only preserves your memories and enables you to create a memoir in any of a variety of forms and formats, but it also provides a basic format from which to organize your recollections. You may or may not want to organize the material in chronological order. Give yourself permission to be creative and self-expressive. This is your record and will become a treasure and a legacy for your family and for your unborn descendants. And you will have the repeated opportunity to enjoy your life in review.

LIFE BOOK

Your Life Book is a documented compilation that contains the accumulated memorabilia of your lifetime and provides a framework for your recollected experiences in a visual format. It is an updated version of the old-fashioned scrapbooks we had as teenagers and can accompany any written record or verbal record you create. In high school I had several such scrapbooks filled with saved pressed flowers from proms, notes from friends, drawings, and assorted papers. As a young adult, I saved Playbills, ticket stubs, and matchbooks of all the restaurants in Manhattan where I had enjoyed meals and kept them in a special box. While it was always a pleasure to revisit them at various times of my life, they remained hidden away and often forgotten. Then the pandemic came and with it the curtailing of most activities. Finally, there was time and space to assemble all I had accumulated over the decades. As I began to reconstruct my life journey, this extremely meaningful activity eased the stress of that difficult time. Little did I realize how much it would continue to mean to me in the years to come as I revisit it from time to time.

Select photos from the various phases of your life to interweave with the memorabilia into the visual record of your Life Book. I used an oversized colorful scrapbook with paper pages where I could paste the pictures and the memorabilia. I subsequently combined them with references to the cultural highlights of that year. In addition to the visual record, I included the names of songs, movies, important legislation, and historical events of that period of time to create a context of the time. Remember to keep adding to your life story in the years to come. Your Life Book will also be a legacy that will speak to descendants you may never come to know.

CELEBRATION OF WISDOM CEREMONY

In the Jewish Renewal tradition, a passage of life ceremony has been added to celebrate seniors transitioning to a new stage of life. Called a *Simchat Chochmat* or Celebration of Wisdom, this ritual addresses an important but often overlooked life passage. According to Rabbi Debra Orenstein, "Such ceremonies offer elders the opportunity to acknowledge a new stage in their lives, and the community an opportunity to honor and learn from them." This basic format can be replicated and celebrated in a variety of ways in a variety of traditions. You can create for yourself and your community a similar ritual designed within your religious, spiritual, or communal framework.

On my 65th birthday, I celebrated my transition to elderhood with a ritual passage ceremony witnessed by family, peers, friends, and cohorts in the beautiful garden of Chochmat Ha Lev, a Jewish Renewal Center in Berkeley, California. The event began with me literally passing through an arched trellis doorway symbolizing my journey from past to future and from middle age to elder. A spiritual leader in my tradition spoke about this life passage followed by each of the guests in turn giving meaningful insights into our relationship and their experience of my spiritual growth. When finished speaking, each received a cut flower symbolizing the fragility and fleeting nature of our lives. At the end of the ceremony, they all received spirit stone sculptures that I had created from stones gathered from sacred places I had visited over the years. Thus, each guest received something valuable and more lasting from the experience that was ephemeral.

After sharing my reflections regarding my own experiences of the passage, we all enjoyed a delicious meal and soothing music.

EMBRACE THE PROCESS

The secret to eldering is to surrender, to slow down, and to simplify. For me, there was no choice. The pandemic stopped all activities, all socializing, all interactions as we had known them and offered no alternative. Resistance was futile. There was nothing anyone could do to change the shutdown. The only choice was to use the time to discover or create another way of being in the world. The quiet and the absence of stimulation provided me, and many others, with an opportunity and the space to adapt in ways not available earlier. It was in that space that this book was born. My pattern had been to always be on the go and suddenly that was no longer possible as a discharge of energy and a mode of expression. The way it once was, was irretrievably gone. And it continues to be that way with no choice but to be open to the way things are now since they will never go back to the way they were.

VISUALIZE THE FUTURE YOU WANT TO CREATE

The best way to create the future you want is to imagine it in full detail. Start with setting aside time to delve deeply and imagine how you would like your best life to be at some specified future date. Visualize the mental images you want to manifest in the coming months. The clearer you are, the easier it will be to orchestrate your vision into your reality. The more you repeat this process in your mind, the stronger the mental imprint and the stronger the new neural pathway.

Your results are even better when you have an actual vision board of images in your mind. Placed in a prominent position, the vision board is a constant reminder of what you are holding in your mind and your heart. Made of heavy stock paper, it displays assembled pictures and printed statements, either handwritten or cut from magazines, which show images or concepts of what you want to create in your life. My last vison board showed prominent pictures of Turkey and Morocco, two countries I just visited.

This device has been used by many famous people including Jack Canfield of *Chicken Soup for the Soul* fame. In fact, in the movie *The Secret,* he showed a picture he had pasted on a vision board many years ago of a house he wanted and then showed a picture of the house he was now living in. It was virtually the same. Of course, remember to be careful what you wish for!

DISCOVER WHAT MAKES YOU HAPPY AND DO MORE OF IT

It is imperative that you discover and pursue what has meaning and value to you because that is what will bring you joy. The happier you are, the higher your vibrations will be and the higher your vibrations are, the more you can shed your light to the world. Therefore, it behooves you to make your vibrations as high as possible because then, not only are you experiencing the joy, but you are spreading it to those around you who could benefit from your glow. A corollary is to do less of what makes you unhappy, anxious or brings you down.

It is not frivolous to be joyous. Rather, it is good for your health. It is good for your state of mind, and it is good for the people around you. So, take heed of Joseph Campbell's advice to, "Follow your bliss" and allow yourself to express your joy without self-consciousness. And you will truly bring more joy to the world.

I wish us all a blissful journey through the remaining years of our lives and like Helen Mirren, "I'd like the last chapter of my life to be like a good read. You get to the end and are sorry to finish."

Hopefully, you will feel the same way about this book, which has been written with love and caring to support a deeper, more meaningful, and more joyous rest of your life. Wishing you a wonderful journey on your way to incorporate what you have learned into a daily practice yielding you abundant health and happiness in the context of Joy.

APPENDIX B
THE "A" GAME

ATTITUDE – is the most significant variable in your entire life. It is also the one thing totally under your control. The late Viktor Frankl, author of *Man's Search for Meaning* realized when in a Nazi concentration camp that no matter how many freedoms were taken away, his attitude was still under his control. He later wrote, "Everything can be taken from a man but one thing: the last of human freedoms—to choose one's attitude in any given circumstances to choose one's own way."

ALLOWING – is the essential first step in relinquishing resistance to your current reality. Since what you resist persists, without allowing what is to be, the game is over.

ACCEPTING – is the next step of coming to terms with precisely those elements in your life that are the most difficult for you to deal with.

ACCOMMODATING – is adjusting your actions and expectations to allow for new possibilities.

APPRECIATION – is looking for the good in everything including things that do not appear to be positive and knowing it is for your best in the long run, if not now.

ADAPTABILITY – involves strategically taking your "A" Game into the world with the recognition that some things can be molded more easily to your liking than others and that some things you cannot change no matter how hard you try. Remembering The Serenity Prayer, you recognize what you can change and accept what you cannot change. Adaptability provides the flexibility to make the necessary shifts when life is unbending.

ACTION – is the only way to make change or progress. After evaluating how to respond to circumstances with which you have been dealt, determine next steps for new results.

APPENDIX C
THE DREADFUL Ds

DOUBT – can grow in your mind, sabotage your intention and your ability to meet your goals.

DISCOURAGEMENT – comes from falsely believing that what you want is not possible when it well might be.

DEPRESSION – is the end result of draining your energy and destroying your dreams.

DISAPPOINTMENT – is an emotional letdown when what was wanted does not manifest. By fixating on what didn't transpire, you do nothing to change the situation, only lament it.

DYSFUNCTIONAL – is that disabling and self-destructive behavior keeping you stuck.

DETACHMENT – is the psychological mechanism that distances you from painful feelings of disappointment, depression, defeat, and despair.

DEFEAT – is the experience of giving up on yourself and all possibilities for change.

DESPAIR – is a deep, dark, depressed mood that impedes any possibility for positive action.

DETERIORATION – is the result of not taking positive action on your own behalf.

DISTANCING – separates you from the flow of life by withdrawing from the world, which only reinforces what you want to eliminate.

DEATH ORIENTATION – is totally giving up on yourself and life itself.

At any point, you can choose to change any and all of these attitudes and attributes and reengage in ways that create new opportunities for less stress and more success.

APPENDIX D
THE RESILIENT Rs

Attributes that will carry you forward because they refresh, reenergize, and reawaken your spirit.

REVIEW – Reviewing your past gives you an opportunity to reconsider old interpretations and make a present time division between what was then and what is now. Then you can choose where it serves you best to put your attention on your goal to redesign your life going forward.

REFRAME – Being able to examine the point of view creates space for greater understanding and a broader perspective. This is one of the basic fundamentals for personal growth.

REAFFIRM – When cherished values, interests, activities, relationships, and beliefs are still a good fit, you are reaffirming that you are at peace with who you are and how you want to live your life.

RECHARGE – Self-care and restorative activities that regenerate your energy and enhance your sense of well-being bring a higher level of energy to your activities.

RENEW – Bringing fresh energy to a relationship, an enterprise, a mindset creates opportunities for self-expression that enables you to continually grow into your best self.

REVITALIZE – Staying present and releasing the past opens the way to the future in new and unanticipated ways since you are no longer tethered to what has been holding you back.

RESILIENCE – Being able to bounce back and rebound is an important trait to be cultivated as it is resilience that brings you back to center and restores balance to your life. Like the child's weighted plastic clown, no matter how much life knocks you down, you bounce back up.

BIRTH IS A BEGINNING
– Rabbi Alvin Fine

Birth is a beginning
And death a destination.
And life is a journey:
From childhood to maturity
And youth to age;
From innocence to awareness
And ignorance to knowing;
From foolishness to discretion
And then, perhaps, to wisdom;

From weakness to strength
Or strength to weakness-
And, often, back again;
From health to sickness
And back, we pray, to health again;

From offense to forgiveness,
From loneliness to love,
From pain to compassion,
And grief to understanding-
From fear to faith;

From defeat to defeat to defeat
Until, looking backward or ahead,
We see that victory lies
Not at some high place along the way,
But in having made the journey,
stage by stage,
A sacred pilgrimage.
Birth is a beginning
And death a destination
And life is a journey,
A sacred pilgrimage-
To life everlasting.

ACKNOWLEDGMENTS

Special thanks to the many people who have contributed their time, expertise and advice to making this book the best it could be, with special recognition to:

Barry Barken – for sharing his personal experience and his inspiring contribution to the field of aging.

Michael Bauer – for his unwavering responsiveness and deep words of wisdom.

Dorothy Bell – editor extraordinaire whose early developmental input has made the book better than it would otherwise have been.

Ella Budovskaya – whose support and suggestions were seminal to the development of this book.

Chip Conley – for highlighting a stage of life in order to support the people in it and doing so with such warmth, wit and good humor.

Michael Larsen – for generously sharing his enormous trove of literary knowledge.

Suzy Prudden – for her generosity in consistently sharing her expertise and being an energetic example of entrepreneurial determination in her senior years.

Barbara Rodgers – for her example of how to live an active engaged life on all levels in her later years as well as for contributing her profound communication skills.

Geoffrey Shaskan – whose unique insights into the content of the book made an important impact into how the story was told.

Janica Smith of PublishingSmith – whose reliability, competence, and good nature made publishing this book (and my earlier book *Climbing the Sacred Ladder: Your Path to Love, Joy, Peace, and Purpose*) a total pleasure.

And to all who made the physical form of this book a reality, with special appreciation to Nick Zelinger for his enormous creativity, which resonated so well with my vision of the book.

Thank you to the Beta Readers for their invaluable feedback and their valuable contribution to the optimal development of this book.

Kate Evans
Ernestine Fields
Heather Hunter
Barbara Rodgers
Geoffrey Shaskan
Hannelore Scheffler
Wanda Whitaker

Dear Reader,
I hope you enjoyed reading
From OY to JOY.
I would greatly appreciate you
posting a review on my Amazon page.

ABOUT THE AUTHOR

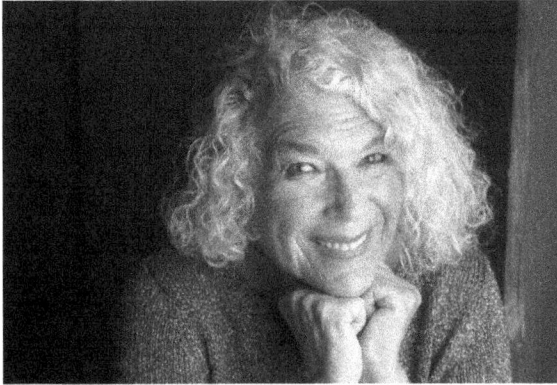

Photographer: Raymond Holbert

Shulamit Sofia is a modern elder with many decades of therapeutic experience in supporting others. She has a BA in psychology from the University of Pennsylvania, a Master's degree in clinical social work from Columbia University, as well as post graduate training with The National Institute of Mental Health in personality development and community consultation. A spiritual seeker since childhood, she has also received training in meditation and mystical practices.

Her academic studies, clinical experience, and spiritual training have enhanced her own life passage and prepared her to support and guide those facing internal and external obstacles in their journey through life. She has learned many lessons along the way, which are now available to you to learn as successful strategies for dealing with life's difficulties.

A lifelong writer, her first book, *Climbing the Sacred Ladder: Your Path to Love, Joy, Peace, and Purpose,* received acclaim from nationally recognized spiritual leaders of all religious dominations. When faced with the pandemic's disruption of her busy life and forced to socially isolate, she returned to writing. Her second book, *From OY to JOY: A Soul Journey to Making the Best of Your Life for the Rest of Your Life,* reflects her own journey and offers guidance to support those dealing with the challenges of aging.

Connect with the author at
https://spiritualaging.org